MAKING THE

*E*STROGEN

DECISION

Also by Gretchen Henkel:
Marketing Your Clinical Practice—Ethically, Effectively, Economically (with Dr. Neil Baum)

MAKING THE
ESTROGEN
DECISION

Gretchen Henkel

LOWELL HOUSE
Los Angeles
CONTEMPORARY BOOKS
Chicago

A A24432

Library of Congress Cataloging-in-Publication Data
Henkel, Gretchen.
    Making the estrogen decision / Gretchen Henkel.
      p.   cm.
    Includes bibliographical references and index.
    ISBN 1-56565-005-0
    1. Menopause—Hormone therapy.   2. Menopause—Hormone therapy—
Complications.   3. Menopause—Popular works.   4. Estrogen—Therapeutic
use.   5. Estrogen—Therapeutic use—Complications.
I. Title.
RG186.H46   1992
618.1'75061—dc20   92-20396
                                                                        CIP

Requests for such permissions should be addressed to:
Lowell House
2029 Century Park East, Suite 3290
Los Angeles, CA 90067

Publisher: Jack Artenstein
Executive Vice-President: Nick Clemente
Vice-President/Editor-in-Chief: Janice Gallagher
Design: Tanya Maiboroda

Manufactured in the United States of America
10 9 8 7 6 5 4 3 2 1

Dedicated to
My husband Richard and my son Jesse,
who give me endless joy and love—
and the time to work

Contents

. . .

Contents

Acknowledgments

• • •

It means so much to have all these bright and supportive people on my "team." I am especially grateful to: Laura Golden Belotti, who does a "clean" edit and was a wonderful cheerleader; Rachel Ross-Pimenta and Ann Snowhook for their fearless forays into the catacombs of UCLA's Biomedical Library; Deborah Anne Lott for her cogent comments and emotional support; Shirley Miyamoto for her insights and attention to detail; Kaliko Orion for her tireless and enthusiastic transcription; Neil Baum, M.D., who shared the "glory" as well as the work of his book; all my friends, who understood when I couldn't see them and who listened to my complaints; my brothers and sisters, for rooting for me all the way; and to two other very special groups of people:

the many women who shared so openly with me their stories about menopause and aging (Margie, Freda, "Mary," "Joanne," "Sophia," and others—you know who you are);

and the following physicians and researchers, who took the time to share their information and expertise with me:

Karen Blanchard, M.D., Assistant Clinical Professor, Department of Obstetrics and Gynecology, UCLA Center for the Health Sciences, and physician in private practice, Women's Medical Group of Santa Monica

Alfred Dashe, M.D., Tarzana, California

Gloria Frankl, M.D., Southern California Permanente Medical Group, Los Angeles, California

R. Don Gambrell, Jr., M.D., Clinical Professor of Endocrinology and Obstetrics and Gynecology, Medical College of Georgia

Sonia Hamburger, Clinical Instructor, Department of Reproductive Medicine, UCSD School of Medicine, La Jolla, California, and Coordinator, Menopause Clinic for Education

Charles Hammond, M.D., Professor and Chairman, Department of Obstetrics and Gynecology, Duke University

John Patrick Holden, M.D., Fellow in Reproductive Endocrinology, Infertility, and Gynecology, UCSD Medical Center, San Diego, California

Winnie Holzman, screenwriter and creator of "Life Class" episode of *thirtysomething,* MGM/Pathé Communications Co.

Howard L. Judd, M.D., Professor of Obstetrics and Gynecology, UCLA, and Executive Director, Division of Reproductive Endocrinology, UCLA and Cedars-Sinai Medical Center, Los Angeles

Carolyn Kaplan, M.D., Assistant Clinical Professor, UCLA, Women's Medical Group, Santa Monica, California

Lewis Kuller, Dr.P.H., Professor and Chairperson, Department of Epidemiology, Graduate School of Public Health, University of Pittsburgh

Susan Lange, O.M.D. (Doctor of Oriental Medicine), Meridian Center, Santa Monica, California

Robert Lindsay, M.D., Ph.D., Professor of Clinical Medicine, Columbia University, New York, and Chief of Internal Medicine, Helen Hayes Regional Bone Center, New York

Daniel W. Nixon, M.D., Atlanta, Georgia

Saar Porrath, M.D., Director, Women's Breast Center, Santa Monica, California, and The Mammography Center, Burbank, California

John P. Rodino, Ph.D., Director, Bionutritional Consultants, Westminster, California

Leon Speroff, M.D., Professor of Obstetrics and Gynecology, Oregon Health Sciences University, Portland

Cynthia A. Stuenkel, M.D., Assistant Clinical Professor of Medicine and Reproductive Medicine, UCSD School of Medicine

Lynn Winters, Ed.D., Graduate School of Education, UCLA

Sidney M. Wolfe, M.D., Director, Public Citizen Health Research Group, Washington, D.C.

Janet Zand, O.M.D. (Doctor of Oriental Medicine), Lic. Ac. (Licensed Acupuncturist), Pacific Palisades, California

Harry K. Ziel, M.D., Southern California Permanente Medical Group, and Emeritus Clinical Professor, Obstetrics and Gynecology, USC School of Medicine

Foreword

· · ·

The number of women entering menopause in our society is increasing rapidly. We now have the largest population of women in history set to enter this phase of life. Between now and the year 2000, according to the U.S. Census Bureau's Department of Projections, there will be 15 million women turning 50 (the average age of menopause is 50-51). This is in addition to the 35 million U.S. women currently over the age of 50. The largest increase will occur in 1997, when 1.9 million women, who were born in 1947 and signaled the beginning of the "baby boom" generation, will turn 50.

This population explosion is being accompanied by an information explosion. Magazines, novels, and self-help books discuss all aspects of menopause, including sexuality and other formerly taboo subjects. Medical information is also increasing rapidly. With the realization that there are health concerns limited to the menopausal woman, the evaluation and management of menopause has become part of mainstream medical practice. Furthermore, funding for menopause research has now become more available. The Women's Health Initiative, funded by the National Institutes of Health, will, over the next several years, direct important research monies to women's health issues. This new recognition and funding have occurred, in part, because more women are entering the upper echelons of health care policymaking and medical research.

Unfortunately, even with greater funding, the answers to all our questions about menopause and its effects on a woman's physiology will not be available for some time. For instance, we know that estrogen supplements help prolong a woman's life by preventing heart disease and loss of bone, but we do not yet fully understand the mechanisms by which the hormone achieves these effects. Until we have more definitive answers, it behooves patients to stay abreast of current developments in this field, and to become partners in their own health care decisions. Ms. Henkel has done a thorough job of addressing the major issues surrounding hormone replacement therapy, and women can take much valuable information from it. Reading *Making the Estrogen Decision* is an excellent way for women to become more involved in their own health care.

Carolyn Kaplan, M.D.

Women's Medical Group of Santa Monica,
Assistant Clinical Professor, UCLA School of Medicine,
Center for Health Sciences, Los Angeles, California

MAKING THE

*E*STROGEN

DECISION

Introduction

Why Is the Estrogen Decision So Important?

• • •

"Estrogen replacement therapy (ERT) probably is the fountain of youth for postmenopausal patients today."
—JEROME ABRAMS, M.D., M.P.H.,
of Robert Wood Johnson Medical School
(part of the University of Medicine and Dentistry,
New Jersey), writing in *New Jersey Medicine*,
March 1991

"Female replacement hormones may someday be remembered as the most recklessly prescribed and dangerous drugs of this century."
—SIDNEY M. WOLFE, M.D., AND RHODA
DONKIN JONES, *Women's Health Alert*

1

No other women's health issues (except, perhaps, hysterectomy and abortion) incite as much controversy in the medical community as whether or not to prescribe estrogen replacement therapy. And when physicians disagree as radically as the above statements illustrate, it can be confusing for women who are trying to make intelligent decisions about their own health and well-being.

As I began the research on this book, I kept hearing in my mind the words my mother's generation used to describe menstruation and menopause. One of my aunts referred to her "friend" who had come to visit, meaning she was having her period. Even among my friends, it wasn't all that unusual to hear that infamous expression, "the curse." I can also remember a girlfriend's mother starting to cry and the other neighborhood mothers talking in hushed tones about her going through "the change."

My mother was the exception to this. As a registered nurse, she wanted my sisters and me to have the correct words to describe what was happening as we grew. After spending several years writing about health and medical topics, intent on being as scientifically correct as possible, I still shrink from using euphemisms to define bodily processes. But now I'm tempted to go back to words like "my friend" and "the change," because they do seem to supply meanings that are lost if you refer to menopause simply as the clinical occurrence of "ovarian failure."

Whether dreaded or welcomed, menopause does indeed represent great change in a woman's life. It's not only the start of another whole phase of her existence, but the loss of estrogen can have far-reaching physical consequences.

My friend Carol looks forward to menopause: "I'll be glad to be finished with this reproductive business," she says, meaning her period. But I have never minded it much. I always welcomed my period, and was nearly 40 before I had my son, so this "reproductive business" has been very precious to me. Now that I'm 44, I find myself thinking about the next stage of my life—all those years when I will not be producing estrogen—and the quality of those years. Researching this book has convinced me that as I grow older, I owe it to myself to stay informed and weigh very carefully my own benefit-risk ratio.

For this book, then, I have talked with doctors on both sides of the hormone replacement therapy (HRT) controversy, as well as those in between. Many physicians recommend it almost unconditionally, hailing it as the "fountain of youth" for postmenopausal women. Others are critical, citing studies that show increased risk of certain types of cancer with the therapy, and decrying hormone replacement therapy as unnatural, an impediment to the normal changes in a woman's life. Interestingly, these physicians' opinions did not necessarily align with their gender. I found both male and female physicians and epidemiologists who are adamantly opposed to giving women estrogens, while many female gynecologists and reproductive endocrinologists are equally adamant in endorsing it. I have also talked with women for and against— women who are just beginning HRT, with much trepidation; women who have decided against it; women who have been on the therapy for 20 years or more. All of this knowledge is presented in the hope that you will benefit from their stories and insights.

Estrogen or hormone replacement therapy is recommended for many women, for a variety of conditions and risk factors. Historically, the most common indication for estrogen has been to relieve the symptoms of menopause, such as hot flashes and vaginal dryness. However, HRT is increasingly prescribed for the menopausal or postmenopausal woman who is at risk for osteoporosis or heart disease. The stories in this book also tell of women who have faced the decision for other reasons: surgical menopause (hysterectomy or oophorectomy [oh-oh-for-EK-tomy]—removal of the ovaries only), amenorrhea (absence or abnormal cessation of menstruation), early menopause, and so on. For each of these women, as for you, the decision has required a careful weighing of benefit versus risk.

Estrogen's Role in Your Health

Why all this emphasis on one hormone? In reality, estrogen is a generic term for a family of estrus-producing sex steroids. Unless otherwise stated, "estrogen" usually refers to the most potent compound of the group, estradiol. Produced primarily in the ovaries by ripening egg follicles, estrogen is critical to the timing of your reproductive cycle. It is also responsible for secondary female sex characteristics, such as development of breasts and lubrication of the vagina. This female sex hormone is beneficial to you in other ways:

- It keeps HDL (high-density lipoprotein) levels high. This is good news for keeping the arteries clear of plaque, deposits that can lead to clogged arteries and heart attack.

- It helps bone to renew itself. Some preliminary studies have shown that estrogen may act directly on

4

the bone, binding to estrogen receptors that stimulate the bone to grow.

- It may protect against the development of rheumatoid arthritis.

You are born with about two million potential eggs in your ovaries. That number diminishes throughout childhood, and the 30 years or so that you menstruate use up most of the remaining number. The eggs that are left eventually dissolve into the ovarian tissue.

Menopause is sometimes defined clinically as the cessation of menstruation for one year. It may help to think of menopause in more functional terms: Your ovaries simply run out of eggs and are no longer able to produce estrogen. (There are other sources of estrogens in your body, however. The steroids androstenedione and testosterone, which also occur naturally in the body, are converted by some tissues into a weaker form of estrogen called estrone. In some women, especially those who tend toward obesity, estrogen derived from extraglandular production can sustain breast fullness and prevent atrophy of the urethra and vagina; but it still may not be enough to make up for the ovarian production levels of the hormone that could protect against osteoporosis and heart disease.)

Living Beyond the Menopause

Until the turn of the century, women did not live substantially beyond their reproductive years. But since 1900, longevity for

5

everyone has increased. Today a woman can expect to live at least 30 and perhaps 40 years beyond menopause. There are 35 million women over 50 in the U.S. By the year 2010, according to estimates by the U.S. Census Bureau's Department of Projections, there will be more than *50 million* women over the age of 50 in the United States alone.

As doctors and researchers are beginning to point out, this large percentage of menopausal and postmenopausal women is a potential public health problem of enormous proportions. That's because when women reach the end of their reproductive lives, their health is at greater risk than men's. Following menopause, women experience bone loss at a faster rate because of estrogen depletion. The rates of loss vary, but most researchers agree that a woman can lose between 2% and 3% of her total bone mass each year in the first five to seven years after menopause. After that time, the rate of bone loss tends to level out. The loss of bone can lead to osteoporosis, in which bone becomes porous and brittle, making a woman more prone to hip, wrist and vertebral fractures. Interestingly, although they too can suffer from age-related osteoporosis, men do not undergo such rapid losses of bone density. The male hormone, testosterone, helps to keep bone strong; it is produced throughout a man's lifetime, tapering off slowly as he ages. Also, men tend to have denser bones to start with than women do.

Following menopause, a woman's risk of heart disease can quickly equal that of a man's her age. Without the protective effects of estrogen, the risk of coronary artery disease increases. Researchers still aren't sure why this is true. It may be because estrogen tends to increase HDL cholesterol levels, but it may also be related to some direct effect that estrogen has on the heart.

Hormone Replacement Therapy (HRT)— Should You or Shouldn't You?

The benefits of taking estrogen after menopause are pretty well established by now: a 50% to 60% decrease in hip and arm fractures brought on by osteoporosis when both estrogen and calcium are taken; and a 50% to 70% reduction in the risk of coronary artery disease, a major cause of heart attacks.

If you looked simply at the conditions estrogen replacement therapy protects against, then the path would be clear-cut. What woman wouldn't want to retard, or prevent altogether, the development of osteoporosis and coronary artery disease? What woman wouldn't want to diminish hot flashes and the resultant loss of sleep? And since estrogen increases blood flow to the vagina and bladder, it also aids in sexual pleasure and bladder toning and control.

If HRT is indeed a "fountain of youth" for postmenopausal women, then why isn't it more generally advocated? Some experts maintain that there is a lack of awareness among patients and physicians of HRT's benefits. However, the risks of HRT are real, just as well known, and perhaps better publicized: increased risk of endometrial and breast cancer, gallstones, and thrombophlebitis.

Physicians and patients alike have been understandably reluctant to embark on a course of hormone replacement that entails such risks. However, in the last 20 years or so, since birth control pills have been in use, science has had more opportunity to study the effects of estrogen on the body. Because estrogen acts as a growth hormone to the endometrium, or lining of the uterus, the longer *unopposed estrogens* (oral or injected estrogen without any other hormone) are given, the higher the risk that a woman will get endometrial cancer.

Researchers conducting epidemiological studies made this connection when they noticed that rates of endometrial cancer went up markedly following the widespread use of estrogens from the mid-1960s to the early 1970s. In response to that data, estrogen is now combined with a progestin (synthetic progesterone) for hormone replacement therapy in women with an intact uterus. (During their reproductive years, women are usually protected from endometrial cancer by progesterone secreted by the corpus luteum, the yellowish casing that forms within a ruptured follicle from the ovary. Release of progesterone triggers regular menstrual bleeding and the sloughing off of the extra uterine growth.) Currently estrogen is also given in a quarter the former dosage—the average dose now is 0.625 mg a day, as opposed to 2.5 mg. In addition, adding progestin to the monthly regimen mimics the body's own menstrual cycle, telling the lining of the uterus to stop growing and to shed itself, resulting in monthly bleeding.

So it appears that hormone replacement therapy is safer than it used to be, even though it is still unclear whether HRT increases a woman's chances of getting breast cancer. And researchers have also noticed that adding progestins to the hormone regimen may adversely affect the blood cholesterol level. But as women's health issues become more of a priority, ongoing studies keep searching for the right dosages and hormones to achieve optimum results.

Until we have more definitive recommendations, the question remains: If you are about to go through menopause, should you consider hormone replacement therapy?

There is no single course of action that will work for every woman. Ultimately, each woman must make the estrogen decision for herself. But you can't do that until you understand the benefits and risks of estrogen replacement therapy.

It is my hope that this book, in conjunction with a caring and competent physician, will help you make your own decision.

1

Estrogen's Role in Your Health

• • •

Sophia, age 57, had resisted taking estrogen for years, even though her doctor had carefully explained all the benefits and risks to her. "I just didn't want to have those extra hormones in my body," she recalls. Sophia elected to take calcium supplements instead, which unfortunately gave her kidney stones. So finally, after two years of tingling under the skin in her arms, legs, and feet ("What I call my itchies"), she listened to her doctor's advice: In all probability this symptom would be much reduced, if not eradicated, if she were to start estrogen replacement therapy. In addition, she'd get the added benefit of protection against osteoporosis, for which she, as a thin Caucasian woman who had smoked for 20 years, was more at risk. Sophia reluctantly agreed to give it a try. It's been eight months now, and she says the difference is like night and day. "If I forget to take

*my pill for two or three days, I can feel my itchies
coming back, and that reminds me to take the
pills. In another two to three days, the tingling is
completely gone again!"*

You may not have reasons as clear-cut as Sophia's for
estrogen replacement therapy. You may even wonder,
"Why is it important to make a decision about estrogen?" or,
"Isn't it dangerous? I've heard it causes cancer," or, "Is it really
necessary to replace a hormone that my body is no longer
making?" Sorting out the range of medical opinions can indeed
be confusing. Some health practitioners claim there are ways
to counterbalance the loss of estrogen after menopause (or
hysterectomy) with what they call more "natural" methods,
such as nutritional supplements, herbal remedies containing
plant estrogens, or acupuncture. On the other hand, many
physicians argue in favor of estrogen therapy not just for
short-term alleviation of menopausal symptoms, but for the
long-term better quality of life that a woman can enjoy.

"There are some patients who come to me with a
challenge," says reproductive endocrinologist Carolyn
Kaplan, M.D., of Women's Medical Group in Santa Monica,
California. "They say, 'I'm in menopause but there's no way
you're going to get me to take that estrogen.' Certainly I'm not
about to twist somebody's arm, but what I try to do is educate
people, and let them decide for themselves which is the right
benefit-risk ratio. For the woman at risk for osteoporosis, there
is an increased risk of hip and forearm fracture if she doesn't
use hormone replacement therapy, and serious fractures probably lead to more deaths than breast cancer does. If a 70-year-
old woman has to have surgery to repair a hip fracture and then
is bedridden during recovery, she has an increased risk of

contracting life-threatening pneumonia. Even in women who remain free of life-threatening fractures, vertebral compression from osteoporosis can lead to chronic debilitating back pain. So I think it's really a matter of quality of life."

There's also the question of a woman's quality of life over a long period of time. Today, many more women are living two to three, even four, decades after menopause, a trend that has been on an increase since the turn of the century, when the average female life expectancy was about 50. The U.S. Census Bureau's Department of Projections puts the expected number of American women over 50 (the average age of menopause) at 52.9 million by the year 2010. That many women who are postmenopausal will have enormous impact on public health issues. These demographics require that we begin now to ask a whole series of questions: Who should get estrogen replacement therapy, if anyone? Is it absolutely indicated? What are the risks? What are the benefits?

The answers to those questions will be different for every woman. Making the decision is a matter of weighing the pluses and minuses of this treatment, as well as finding out about its long-term effects. Unfortunately, all the long-term effects won't be known for several years yet. For instance, the PEPI (or Postmenopausal Estrogen/Progestin Interventions) Trial won't be completed until mid-1994 or early 1995. Now being conducted at seven U.S. medical universities, that study focuses on the effects of combined estrogen and progestin therapy on blood cholesterol levels. In addition to other factors, such as effect on insulin levels, researchers are looking for the optimum combination of estrogen and progestin that will eliminate monthly bleeding (which makes HRT unpleasant for some women) and will not adversely affect the good cholesterol levels. The study's secondary objectives are to evaluate treatment effects on other lipids, bone loss, uterine wall changes, blood pressure, and quality of life. Even when that study is published, researchers still won't know about estrogen's direct effects, if any, on the heart itself.

Other studies, such as those conducted by Lila E. Nachtigall, M.D., since the early 1970s on the link between osteoporosis and estrogens, have been much more definitive. In fact, there's now enough information for physicians to routinely recommend HRT as a preventative against this crippling chronic disease. And there's a side benefit to all this research: As investigators study the long-term effects of hormone replacement therapy, they learn even more about the mechanisms of our hormonal systems.

How Does Estrogen Affect You?

Medical science has known about estrogen's role in a woman's reproductive health for some time. There are a number of estrogen-dependent organs in your body: your breasts, uterus, cervix, vagina, and bladder. Scientists are now finding that even more tissues of the body are estrogen receptor-positive, which means that they can bind with and be affected by estrogen as well. Your skin, especially the hair follicles and sebaceous glands, according to reproductive endocrinologist Carolyn Kaplan, M.D., have estrogen receptors. One of the effects estrogen has on skin cells is to encourage them to take up more water, so your skin feels fuller and more resilient with more fluid in the tissues. There are other examples of tissues and systems that respond to estrogen. Through grants from the

National Institutes of Health, much of the present research is concerned with estrogen's effect on bone mass. Estrogen plays a role in helping bone to absorb calcium, thus preventing loss of mass. Without estrogen, the bones of susceptible individuals tend to lose mass and become porous and brittle, increasing the risk of hip, spinal, and forearm fractures. (In Chapter Three you'll learn more about the specific risk factors for osteoporosis, and why women are more likely to get the disease than men.)

Another role for estrogen has to do with raising the levels of HDL (high-density lipoprotein) cholesterol in the blood, and lowering the levels of LDL (low-density lipoprotein). HDL, the so-called "good cholesterol," has the ability to enclose bits of fat and cholesterol inside a high-density "envelope." The fats are thus carried out of the bloodstream instead of breaking down and depositing fatty plaque on artery walls, a dangerous condition that leads to blocked arteries and heart attack. The "bad" cholesterol, LDL, breaks down easily and deposits fats along artery walls. So lowering LDL is another desirable effect of estrogen.

Estrogens have an effect on your nervous system as well. Scientists think the hormone can subtly alter levels of catecholamines, such as dopamine and epinephrine, which act on the nervous system, resulting in mood fluctuations. Estrogen also plays a role in sexual desire, a complex set of hormonal messages and feedback mechanisms between the pituitary, hypothalamus and ovaries. When a woman is having normal ovulatory cycles, the mature follicle tells her ovary to begin turning its naturally occurring androgens (male hormones) into estrogens. The woman's estrogen level rises, and she usually experiences increased sexual receptivity during monthly ovulation.

15

Where Does Estrogen Come From?

When we talk about estrogen we usually think of one hormone, a steroidal compound made primarily in the ovaries when an egg follicle matures. But in fact, there are three estrogen compounds made in the body—estradiol, estriol, and estrone, in descending order of potency. Estradiol, the type produced by the ovary, is part of the complicated feedback system between the hypothalamus, pituitary, and ovary that results in the normal monthly ovulatory cycle. Estrone, a low-level estrogen, is converted from androgens in fatty tissue. The relatively weak estriol is produced as a by-product of estradiol and estrone metabolism.

Men also produce estrogens, but in much smaller quantities—just as women produce certain amounts of the male hormone testosterone in their bodies. It is not so much the presence of a hormone, but its quantity, that determines the sex characteristics of male and female.

There is a continual power struggle between male and female hormones taking place internally. In fact, a woman's ovaries are also an androgen (male hormone)-producing organ. When a woman has normal ovulatory cycles, according to Dr. Kaplan, one follicle in the ovary outpaces growth in the rest of the ovary and manages to turn most of that androgen into estrogen, so that the ratio is balanced in favor of estrogen. After menopause, when there are no more eggs to stimulate conversion of those androgens to estrogens, some women may see an increase in facial hair and oily skin, which are androgenic effects.

Estrogens are universal growth hormones. They occur in other mammals—in fact, the most often prescribed form of estrogen, Premarin, is taken from the urine of pregnant mares.

16

Interestingly, forms of estrogen are also found in certain plants. One milder form of estrogen given to women by naturopathic practitioners is derived from the Mexican yam. Many naturopathic physicians rely on preparations using these plant estrogens, called phyto-estrogens, to deliver a weak estrogen effect to counteract menopausal symptoms. (You'll learn more about alternative treatments in Chapter Six.) Medical researchers often point out that because they are very weak estrogens, phyto-estrogens are not effective in preventing bone loss.

IN THE BEGINNING. While in the uterus, the female fetus has millions of germ cells (potential follicles). From a peak of six to seven million potential eggs at 20 weeks in utero, the eggs begin to diminish in number. They go through the same cycle that they will when a young woman enters puberty: Some follicles form, ripen, and then go through *atresia,* or degeneration, before reaching maturity.

At puberty a young woman has about 300,000 follicles left. At the rate of about 400 a month, these graafian follicles are stimulated by the secretion of FSH (follicle stimulating hormone) by the pituitary. In response to this "nudge" from FSH, the follicles grow. As they grow, the ovary converts the precursor androgen into estradiol. Essentially a growth hormone, this estrogen then stimulates the lining of the uterus to grow and thicken in preparation for receiving a fertilized egg. At a certain point in the monthly cycle, after ovulation, the estrogen is counterbalanced by progesterone, secreted by the corpus luteum (a yellowish mass that forms after the follicle ruptures). The corpus luteum is simply the leftover egg sac which shifts to making progesterone. Its yellowish color comes from the amount of cholesterol it gathers to make progesterone. It is this surge of progesterone that often causes a "puffy" feeling (from water retention) and mood swings. The progesterone then triggers the sloughing off of the uterine lining, causing the menstrual period.

THE CONTINUUM CHANGES. From puberty until a woman's 40s, follicle maturation and estrogen production, followed by degeneration of the egg, continue the monthly cycles (unless, of course, fertilization and pregnancy occur; then another whole string of events takes place). Sometime between ages 38 and 42, ovulation becomes less frequent. Some researchers believe that the follicles left in the ovary at this point are those most resistant to stimulation by gonadotropins, hormones that stimulate the ovaries (such as FSH, follicle stimulating hormone, or LH, luteinizing hormone), and thus are least likely to mature. At any rate, fewer eggs mean less estrogen production, and levels of the hormone gradually begin to diminish.

At midlife, the monthly ovulatory cycle begins to change and a woman's body enters another continuum, that of the menopause. The remaining egg follicles become more and more resistant to stimulation and eventually dissolve into the body's tissue. With a diminishing supply of eggs, the ovary produces less and less estrogen, and the uterine lining begins to thin. Menstrual periods become lighter and for the most part infrequent. Within about a year after the last menstrual period, the ovary no longer produces estrogen. There are other indirect sources of estrogen, such as conversion of fatty tissue into weak, endogenous estrogens. But these levels are not enough to sustain tissues that previously depended upon the hormone for vitality. Because estrogen affects so many tissues and organs in the body, its withdrawal can cause a multitude of symptoms and conditions. This "progressive estrogen withdrawal" is characterized by some of the following general symptoms:

Menstrual periods become generally lighter and usually more infrequent. For some women this is a gradual process, happening along a continuum. For others, the menstrual periods stop abruptly and do not return.

Appearance of hot flushes, also called flashes, which elicit sometimes-profuse perspiration following a sensation of intense body heat. They last anywhere from a few seconds to several minutes, but tend to occur more frequently at night, disrupting sleep. They also happen more frequently during times of stress. Researchers have shown that the hot flash is not related to a conventional release of body heat, like the sweating you experience during a hard physical workout. Rather, the lowered estrogen levels in the body trigger overproduction of other hormones, such as FSH and LH, whose rising levels coincide with the stimulation of the brain's heat release mechanisms. From 75% to 85% of all menopausal women experience this symptom, in varying degrees. Whether or not it is treated with estrogens, it is a symptom that goes away over time—in one to two years for most women, five or more years for others.

Atrophy or shrinking of the mucus-producing tissues in the vagina, as well as skin and bladder tissues; and a flattening of the breasts. These tissues and organs all

19

have estrogen receptors. Without estrogen the vagina becomes drier, making penetration uncomfortable.

Emotional disturbances. It is still not clear whether estrogen withdrawal is directly related to mood swings and emotional difficulties experienced during menopause. One medical textbook points out in a cavalier way that if a woman is well adjusted in her life, she will not have a hard time adjusting to menopause. Other scientists are more discerning. They recognize that emotional disturbances, ranging from increased irritability and anxiety to extreme mood swings, often coincide with menopause. But the disturbances may not be directly caused by the physical changes. In our society, menopause is a loaded time for women. A premium is put on youth and beauty, and women may tend to feel less vital once their bodies give concrete evidence of the aging process. In addition, menopause can be just one more stressor in a life filled with concerns about children leaving home, aging parents, career pressures and more. Interestingly, in Japanese society women do not experience as much emotional difficulty during menopause as American women do. Could this be due to a more respected place for older people in that society?

These are some, but not all, of the immediate effects of estrogen withdrawal. Other effects can include extremely sensitive gums, arthralgia (joint pain), and a general feeling of anxiety. These various symptoms cause great discomfort for some women, but only minor discomfort for others. Hormone replacement therapy is one of the best antidotes medical science has for addressing these symptoms. Almost everyone agrees that HRT is a good idea for menopausal women who are extremely uncomfortable. But because of increased longevity in our society, physicians are also concerned about the long-term effects of estrogen loss, which have more serious consequences:

Loss of bone mass. We begin to lose bone mass beginning at age 35 whether we're male or female, at a rate of about 1% a year. For women, the greatest percentage of loss appears to occur right after menopause. Caucasian and Asian women start losing bone earlier than do black and Latin women. Those women who are thin and/or who are smokers are at even greater risk. (The risk for an ex-smoker—say, one who hasn't smoked in 10 years—is not known.) Without estrogen, the bone loses protein and calcium. Although calcium supplementation and weight-bearing exercise can mitigate some of this bone loss, they cannot prevent it entirely. Instituting estrogen therapy after menopause can improve bone density, as can regular weight-bearing exercise and calcium supplements, but they cannot restore the bone to its former levels of density.

Loss of protective effects in the blood. It is a well-known fact that women up to about age 50 are much less likely to have heart attacks than men. This is because of the protective effects of estrogen against heart disease. Estrogen causes the levels of HDL, or good cholesterol, to rise. The Nurses' Health Study in 1985 demonstrated a 50% reduction in risk of coronary disease among women taking estrogen. The PEPI Trial is now currently studying the effects of HRT on blood lipid levels. This double-blind study (meaning that neither researchers nor participants know which volunteers are taking which hormone replacement or placebo) is using several treatments:

- unopposed estrogen (estrogen given alone)
- estrogen plus a cyclic progestin (a form of progesterone is added the last 10 days of the cycle of pills, to mimic the body's own menstrual cycle)
- estrogen plus a continuous progestin (a small amount of progesterone is given each day, continuously, to avoid the side effect of menstrual periods)
- estrogen and a micronized progesterone (progesterone in a very fine powder)
- a placebo.

All study participants are seen a total of 14 times over a three-year period. They are given physical examinations, blood tests, ECGs (electrocardiograms), bone density studies, biopsies of uterine tissue, mammography, and so on. Researchers are looking for the most beneficial combination of estrogen and progesterone, because with unopposed estrogen (not "interrupted" by progesterone), the uterine lining continues to grow and proliferate and can cause concern about risk of precancerous changes in the uterus.

The effects of estrogen loss are presented not as doomsaying, or to coerce women into initiating hormone replacement therapy. As you will see later in this book, there are many proponents of alternative or naturopathic approaches to dealing with the changes that menopause brings. Hormone replacement therapy may not be a good idea for everyone, and for some women, it is absolutely contraindicated.

When Should You Start Thinking About Estrogen?

The term "menopause" is especially apt, because it signifies bodily processes that do not simply stop—they "pause." Think of the changes of menopause happening on a continuum: Your egg supply is gradually depleted, estrogen production tapers off, you begin to feel your body shifting in a variety of subtle—and not so subtle—ways. Practicing good health habits is wise no matter what age you are. One aspect of self-care is to keep yourself informed and to be aware of your own body's changes. By your mid-40s, you will want to start thinking about the estrogen decision. (It may be earlier, if you have a family history of early menopause.)

Most women see their gynecologist at least once a year for a checkup and Pap smear. That might be the most opportune time to begin talking with your physician about the signposts of menopause and the advisability of estrogen replacement. Ask for recommendations and recent studies the doctor finds particularly helpful; let him or her know your concerns and priorities.

In the following chapters I cover the key concerns about the estrogen decision: the pros and cons, who's most likely to benefit from the therapy, and who should avoid it. Many physicians espouse taking hormones because of their protective effects against osteoporosis and heart disease. But other voices advise caution, because we simply do not know for sure whether estrogens cause breast cancer. Would you be taking too much of a risk if you took estrogen? Would you be foolish *not* to? You'll hear from a variety of experts who'll discuss the current thinking in the medical and alternative healing communities, and learn about steps you can take *now* that will benefit you in the years after menopause. My aim is to help you be better prepared to make your own decision in partnership with your physician.

2

What Is Estrogen Replacement Therapy?

• • •

"I had a hysterectomy 21 years ago, when I was 41. I still had my ovaries, but they gave me the estrogen anyway, because once you lose your uterus, you also lose hormones. I happened to have a very good gynecologist at that time and he and I sat down and talked about estrogen therapy. There was no resistance on my part. I was aware of the protective effects of estrogen, and because I didn't have a uterus, the question of uterine cancer didn't arise.

"I really didn't experience any side effects when I started taking the estrogen. In fact, after the hysterectomy and getting on the Premarin, I realized that I felt more energetic. I had been tired for 20 years and hadn't known it!

"Taking estrogen is one of the best things I've ever done. It has allowed me to continue life without fragile bones and dry mucous membranes, and essentially function in many respects as though I were still of childbearing age."

—ANN, age 62

Each woman is unique. We each have a distinct physical makeup and will go through menopause in a different way. There are many reasons that physicians prescribe estrogen to replace your body's female hormones, and hysterectomy is one of the most common. For whatever reason your gynecologist, internist, or family practitioner might suggest hormone replacement therapy, the ideal scenario is one in which you sit down and have a reasoned discussion about your own health and risk factors.

Ann had no hesitation about taking estrogen. That was probably due to a combination of factors: her own self-education, her trust in her physician, and the fact that all the women on her mother's side of the family had very regular and healthy menstrual cycles. And, she adds, "there is no history of breast cancer in my family, so that has made me much more comfortable about it too."

Throughout this book, you'll learn about a variety of women's experiences with estrogen. And you'll discover information that will help you assess whether HRT might be a good idea for you. This chapter will give you an overview of the methods of giving hormone replacement therapy. I'll list the most commonly prescribed brand-name drugs, their dosages, possible side effects, and drug interactions, as well as the history you should give your doctor. In Chapter Three you'll learn more about who can benefit from HRT. And in later chapters, I'll cover the benefits and risks of the therapy.

Estrogens and progestins are given in several different ways, and for a variety of reasons other than menopause. Most women are familiar with the combination of the two used in oral contraceptives. Both estrogens and progestins are also administered as an adjunct to chemotherapy in some cancers of the breast in women and cancer of the prostate in men.

For the purpose of this book, I'll be focusing the discussion on estrogens and progestins used to restore the hormonal balance that a woman's own body maintains when she is in her reproductive years.

The most common indications for which your physician may suggest hormone replacement therapy to you are:

1) as a treatment for menopausal symptoms (hot flashes, vaginal atrophy and dryness, etc.) and

2) as a prophylactic (preventive) measure to protect against the development of osteoporosis or heart disease.

Some women will experience side effects, others will not. I've talked with women who decided to start HRT but who still feel ambivalent about the therapy because of its long-term effects. Others are grateful they started HRT because it helped them deal with an extremely uncomfortable menopause, and they plan to continue the therapy for a long time.

Estrogen replacement therapy, or ERT, is the replacement of the estrogens your body is no longer producing because of either natural or surgical menopause (hysterectomy or oophorectomy).

As I mentioned in the Introduction, estrogens are most commonly prescribed in the United States as a combination therapy, together with progesterone. This is because giving estrogens alone, or unopposed, can cause an abnormal growth of cells (hyperplasia) in the uterine lining (the endometrium). Hyperplasia, if not diagnosed and treated, can lead to endometrial cancer. However, if a woman no longer has her uterus, the addition of a progestin isn't necessary, as in Ann's case. In rare cases, a woman with an intact uterus may be given estrogen only (usually in very small doses). Some women actually request this therapy, because of adverse reactions to progestin. This type of replacement would be accompanied by regular endometrial biopsies to monitor the effects on the uterine lining. For the most part, though, postmenopausal women who have not had hysterectomies are placed on hormone replacement therapy (HRT) rather than ERT.

Estrogens and progestins are prescription drugs. Given alone or in combination, they introduce a pharmacological substance to your body and should only be taken while under the supervision of your physician. You should always be alert for side effects of *any* drugs you take, whether prescription or over-the-counter. (Even Tylenol or aspirin can cause damage to the liver or stomach if overused.)

If you are on a hormone replacement therapy program, most physicians recommend a thorough annual checkup, which should include a breast exam, Pap smear, complete blood workup (cholesterol levels, glucose levels, clotting factors, etc.), and a mammogram. Some women on HRT see their gynecologist or internist every six months for checkups. It depends on your situation and your doctor's recommendations. (Chapter Nine focuses on recommended tests and commonsense monitoring while on HRT.)

28

In the 1960s and early 1970s estrogens had a reputation as a fountain of youth for postmenopausal women. This led to what some experts now believe was an over-prescription of the drug. By 1975 reports of increased incidence of uterine cancer began to make the headlines, and prescription decreased. In the last 10 to 15 years researchers have worked out much lower dosages, and physicians do not advise a higher dosage than necessary to relieve symptoms, so that the endometrium is not overly stimulated. Lila Nachtigall, M.D., who conducted one of the first controlled, prospective (in which participants are selected in the present and followed into the future), double-blind studies on estrogen replacement therapy (*American Journal of Obstetrics and Gynecology,* January 1979), says in her book *Estrogen* that you should "always take the lowest amount of any drug that will do the job assigned to it." She notes that although Premarin comes in a dosage as low as 0.3 mg, most women require .625 mg to prevent osteoporosis.

Depending on your particular set of circumstances and the reason for the prescription, estrogens may be given orally, in pill form; transdermally, in a patch applied to the skin; or intravaginally, in a cream.

In the past, estrogen was also given in intramuscular injections, but this practice is not common today.

See the figure at the end of this chapter for the various brand names and dosages of estrogen and progestin.

Estrogens

First introduced in 1933, estrogens as a drug class include both natural and synthetic compounds. Estrogens are steroidal compounds, basically growth hormones, and are now given in much lower dosages than they were even in the 1970s. The most common brand names of oral estrogens are Estrace, Estrovis, Ogen, and Premarin. Premarin, manufactured by Wyeth-Ayerst, is probably the most widely prescribed oral estrogen, and contains the conjugated (combined) estrogens from the urine of pregnant mares. Estrace is a synthetic estrogen, called estradiol (es-tra-DYE-all).

How Estrogen Works

When you take estrogens, your body responds in a variety of ways. Certain cells and tissues contain estrogen receptors, to which estrogens can bind. This triggers a complicated biological process in which the cell's protein and nucleic acid synthesis is affected by actions on the nucleus. Most female sex organs, such as the breasts and vagina, are directly affected by estrogen. This accounts for the fact that, in addition to the intermittent or absent menstrual cycle, the two most pronounced symptoms of menopause are a flattening of the breasts and a thinning and drying out of the vagina.

Estrogen also affects a process called *remodeling,* which takes place in the bone marrow. (The process is explained in greater detail in Chapter Three, in the section entitled "Consequences of Bone Loss.") Additionally, when estrogens are metabolized by the liver, they cause a lowering of blood cholesterol levels. Other studies have shown the effects of estrogens on other mucous membranes, such as the lining of the mouth.

How Estrogen Is Given

ORAL ESTROGEN is the way most women get their dosage for hormone replacement therapy. Dosages range from .3 to 1.25 mg for the first 21 to 25 days of the month. Different women require different dosages, but usually the dosage is .625 mg. Typically dispensed in quantities of 100 tablets, the standard .625 mg Premarin dose costs about $33 for 100 tablets, which last about four months. As you'll see later in this section, an additional pill containing progestin is started at about day 13 or day 16 of those 25 days, to stimulate shedding of the uterine lining via a menstrual period.

There are other ways you can take estrogens too:

VAGINAL CREAMS contain anywhere from .01 to .625 mg of estrogens, in either conjugated (biologic combined) or synthetic (chemically produced) form. Brand names include Estraguard, Premarin, Ogen, and Estrace, and a 1½ ounce tube can cost as much as $30. How long it lasts depends on how much you use. Using a vaginal applicator, you insert the estrogen cream directly into your vagina—how often will be at the discretion of your physician, based on what works best to alleviate your symptoms.

Estrogens in cream form are prescribed to deal with the vaginal changes of menopause, such as drying and thinning of the vaginal walls, and the resulting lack of lubrication, which can make intercourse very uncomfortable. Estrogens applied in the vagina can also help tone the bladder, thus preventing incontinence and multiple urinary tract infections.

Doctors caution that even though vaginal creams are topically applied, they do deliver a considerable amount of

31

estrogen to the bloodstream. They should not be used as a lubricant nor applied just before intercourse, because the estrogen can have adverse effects on your partner. A man can experience irritation of the penis—and, if enough gets into his bloodstream, enlargement of his breast tissues! It may be wise to time your applications for mornings or midday if you usually have intercourse in the evening. And since the estrogens in cream form are also capable of stimulating uterine lining growth, an oral progestin may be prescribed to counteract that effect.

TRANSDERMAL means entering *through* the skin. The Estraderm patch, made by Ciba-Geigy, looks like a large, round, transparent Band-Aid, about the size of your palm. You apply this patch, which contains synthetic estradiol, to your abdomen and change it every 3 to 4 days (twice weekly per Ciba-Geigy patient instructions). Estradiol is a strong form of estrogen; it is easily absorbed through the skin and from there enters the bloodstream. The dosage is .05 to 1 mg. A month's supply of Estraderm patches (averaging two a week) ranges in cost from $23 to $28, depending on the dosage of hormone and the pharmacy you use.

According to Dr. Howard L. Judd, a renowned reproductive endocrinologist at UCLA and currently a principal investigator in the NIH's PEPI (Postmenopausal Estrogen/Progestin Interventions) Trial, "Estraderm patch delivers estradiol into your general circulation as the ovary does, so it comes closer to replicating ovarian function than any form of oral estrogen administration."

The advantage to taking estrogen in this way is that oral estrogens are filtered through the liver, and some of the estrogen is converted into by-products that affect other organs. Because it isn't metabolized in the liver, as all oral medications are, transdermal estrogen may result in less risk of hypertension, gallbladder disease and thrombosis. (You may remember these possible risks from taking birth control pills in your 20s.) Moreover, lower dosages (.05 to 0.1 mg) are required. The beneficial effects on bone mass appear to be the same as with oral estrogen, and the clinical symptoms of menopause, including hot flashes, irritability, and poor concentration, are relieved in the same way as with oral estrogens.

However, as Dr. Judd points out, there is still debate about whether this is the best way to take estrogens. For instance, even though it does lower the total blood cholesterol, transdermal estrogen may not cause the HDL ("good") cholesterol to rise. Studies are currently underway to find out whether it is as protective against heart disease as are the oral forms of the drug.

Still, Margie, who's 63, finds the Estraderm patch the most convenient way to take her estrogen. She applies a patch to one side of her abdomen early in the week, then applies a second patch to the opposite side of her abdomen three days later. But while Margie adjusted to the "minor itching" caused by the adhesive in the patch itself, it became a major irritant to Nicky, 64, who had to switch to a pill form of estrogen.

The dosage of estrogen is smaller with a transdermal patch. However, the amount of hormone delivered to your system can still affect your endometrium. So a progestin is additionally prescribed to women with an intact uterus who use a patch, for the same reason that it is given to women who take estrogen orally. The progestin balances the effects of the estrogen on the endometrium.

Side Effects of Estrogens

The potential side effects of taking estrogens include possible weight gain and fluid retention, "breakthrough" bleeding (between periods), altered menstrual patterns, and increased susceptibility to yeast infections. More rarely, some women experience an increased sensitivity to sunlight (photosensitivity), headaches, increased blood pressure, and decreased sugar tolerance.

As with any prescription or over-the-counter drug, estrogens should not be taken by some women. These include women who:

- are pregnant

- have impaired liver function

- have abnormal and/or unexplained vaginal bleeding

- have a history of thrombophlebitis (blood clots in the vein), embolism (sudden blocking of an artery by a clot), or stroke. Although it lowers blood cholesterol levels, estrogen tends to increase blood clotting factors in the blood.

Your physician will do a complete physical and screening before starting you on hormone replacement therapy. This should include taking a complete medical history, if it's not already in your chart. If you have any of the following risk factors, your doctor needs to know:

- *family history of breast cancer.* Current research will be covered in Chapter Four on the risks of HRT. But

34

basically, the jury's still out on this one. Most doctors agree that breast cancer in a first-degree relative (mother, sisters) is a bigger risk to you than a history of breast cancer in a second-degree relative (grandmothers from either side of the family).

- *a previous adverse reaction to estrogens.*
- *history of asthma, kidney problems, liver problems, migraine headaches, epilepsy, or clinical depression.*

It's very important for you to furnish your physician with complete information, stresses John P. Holden, M.D., a fellow in reproductive endocrinology at the University of California, San Diego Medical Center. Are you being treated with other medications? It's important that your doctor know. Medications such as anticoagulants, given to people prone to forming clots, may be less effective in women taking estrogens. Other medications, such as certain corticosteroids given for arthritis, may be *more* effective in the presence of estrogen. Your dosages of either the estrogen or additional medications will be adjusted accordingly. Do you drink alcohol to excess? Do you smoke cigarettes? Do you take any illegal drugs? Some people shy away from discussing these matters with their physicians. To do so deprives you and your doctor of the complete picture needed to make the estrogen decision.

Progestins

Since medical researchers know that unopposed estrogen can lead to precancerous changes in the endometrial lining of the uterus, progestins are the necessary complement to replacement estrogens. Progestins induce menstrual bleeding, during which excess growth of the endometrium is sloughed off. Some researchers believe this monthly period leaves a woman on HRT more resistant to uterine cancer than non-estrogen-taking menopausal women.

How Progestins Work

Because they can alter the endometrium, progestins, when used daily as an oral contraceptive, basically trick the body into thinking that it is already pregnant by inducing and maintaining a uterine lining rich with blood cells. They also suppress the release of FSH (follicle stimulating hormone) by your pituitary so you will not ovulate or stimulate mucus production in your cervix that allows sperm to enter the uterus. Alone or in combination with estrogen, progestins are often used to prevent conception. Progestins are also given to regulate menstrual periods in women whose hormonal imbalances make them irregular or amenorrheic.

In the presence of estrogens, progestins induce withdrawal bleeding within three to seven days of stopping the drug.

How Progestins Are Given

Added to the (typically) 25-day course of the estrogens, progestins also come in pill form. Brand-name preparations are

36

Amen, Curretab, and Provera, and tablets are available in 2.5, 5, and 10 mg strengths. A 100-tablet supply (which should last about 10 months, depending on your regimen) retails for around $40 for the 2.5 mg size, $60 for the 5 mg, and $70 for the 10 mg dosage. Another progestational agent, Megace (Bristol Myers), is another choice used by many gynecologists. A woman takes progestin (the dosage and timing are prescribed by her physician) once a day, beginning at about day 13 of the estrogen, for five to ten days. At the end of that time she will get her menstrual period.

For the progestin part of her therapy, Margie takes Provera for seven days out of the month. "I can never remember which are the *last* seven days of the month," she notes, "so I just take it the first seven days of each month. The doctor said that was fine, and it works to help me take it." This works for Margie because she is using the patch every week, and those seven days she takes Provera correspond to the seven out of 28 days when her body used to make the progesterone. If you are taking oral estrogens, your routine for the progesterone may be different. Some women take oral estrogen daily and oral progesterone the first week to 10 days of the month.

Side Effects of Progestins

When she first started taking Provera, Margie noticed that she began to feel quite moody and "down." The pills she had been prescribed had a line down the middle, so she simply split them and took half of the regular pill. At her next regular checkup, she told her nurse practitioner, "I hope I haven't screwed it up by taking it this way." The nurse practitioner asked whether

her periods had stopped or changed. "No," said Margie. So the nurse practitioner simply prescribed the next lower dose of Provera, and things were fine.

In Margie's case, halving the dosage did not turn out to be a disaster. However, *you should not change your own dosage without first consulting your physician.* If you notice side effects, such as increased emotional upset, anxiety, or bloating, write it down and either call or visit your doctor. The dosage can be adjusted according to your needs.

As Margie noted in her case, depression can be a side effect of progestins. Others include dizziness, headaches, fatigue, fluid retention, premenstrual irritability, and allergic rash. The following are rare but *very serious* effects of this medication. The symptoms are also listed.

RARE EFFECTS OF PROGESTINS

Side Effect	Warning Sign
Liver toxicity	Jaundice—yellowish tinge to skin and eyes
Thrombophlebitis	Pain or tenderness in thigh or leg; may be accompanied by swelling of foot or leg
Pulmonary embolism	Sudden shortness of breath, chest pain, cough, bloody sputum
Stroke	Sudden headache, blackout, weakness, or paralysis of any extremity; severe dizziness, slurred speech

* Source: *The Essential Guide to Prescription Drugs, 1992,* James W. Long, M.D., HarperCollins, New York, 1992. By permission.

You should report any new symptom or side effect to your doctor. Also, there are certain drugs (steroids, antidepressants, the antibiotic rifampin—brand names Rifadin, Rimactane) that may adversely interact with progestins. So if you are currently taking any other medications, make sure to apprise your doctor of this fact. Each woman's system will react differently to various hormones. For some women, like Margie and Patricia, 65, progestins caused more side effects than the estrogen. Margie dealt with it by taking half the regular amount of progestin; Patricia eventually stopped taking the progestin altogether, and went in for regular endometrial biopsies as a safeguard.

Medications can also interact with the absorption of nutrients in your system. Because progestins lower the levels of folates and pyridoxine in the body, you should seek out sources of vitamin B-6 and folic acid in your diet. (You can replenish vitamin B-6 by eating protein-rich meat, liver, poultry, fish, egg yolks, and tomato juice; folic acid is commonly found in fresh green vegetables, whole grains, and dry beans.)

Pills or Patches—Which Is for You?

Women I interviewed for this book had different attitudes about oral and transdermal estrogens. Some found it a hassle to chart the days they were taking estrogen and the days they were to start the progestin. Others very easily incorporated their pill-taking into their daily routine. When you talk with your doctor, he or she may have certain recommendations. But the choice will be yours. And if one method isn't working, you will probably be able to try another. For instance, Laura, age 50, told me that she liked the convenience of the patch but found that even the 0.05 mg dosage was causing her to experience extreme breast tenderness. When she complained about this to her doctor, he suggested that she simply wear one patch a week instead of two, thus effectively cutting the dosage in half. He advised her to change the patch from the left to the right side of her abdomen, to improve absorption into the bloodstream from change of site.

If you forget to take one of your pills, it is not a good idea to double up on your dosage the next day. You could induce nausea or vomiting, and it's not advisable, in general, to introduce a double dose of the hormones into your body. Simply pick up where you left off and continue the regular monthly schedule.

Current Developments and Thinking

It is extremely difficult to estimate how many postmenopausal women are currently on hormone replacement therapy. According to the *Journal of the American Medical Association* (April 17, 1991), the number of estrogen prescriptions dispensed in the United States climbed from 14 million in 1980 to 20 million in 1986. However, it is quite common for women to take hormones just before and after menopause and then to stop taking them. Jane A. Cauley and her colleagues (*American Journal of Obstetrics and Gynecology*, November 1990) found that only 13.7% of 9,704 women age 65 and over were using any type of hormone replacement—estrogen alone or in combination with a progestin. That's a very small percentage of the female postmenopausal population.

The two major reasons women stop taking estrogens, says Leon Speroff, M.D., of Oregon Health Sciences University in Portland, are bleeding and fear of cancer. Researchers across the United States and around the world are studying the possible connection between HRT and breast cancer. (I'll go into that at length in Chapter Four.)

What about the bleeding, though? As long as a woman takes cyclic progestins, there will be some bleeding. Eva, an active, involved 64-year-old woman, doesn't mind the periods. But other women are, understandably, ready to be free of menstrual periods that have been with them since their adolescent years.

There are several current drug trials testing the effectiveness of one pill that combines the estrogens and progestin. The progestin is in a much smaller dose but is given continuously, and after minimal spotting for the first few months, does not create a monthly "period." Such a pill is included in the PEPI Trial, and Dr. Speroff is also involved in drug studies using new products by Wyeth-Ayerst and Parke/Davis. In addition, there's a new patch by Parke/Davis that would be put on once a week rather than every three days. "All the pharmaceutical companies are jumping into this," says Dr. Speroff, "because they see the enormity of the market and they're all looking to develop combined products."

The important factor that still has to be decided is how these progestins affect blood cholesterol. We know that estrogens lower the cholesterol level and essentially increase the level of good cholesterol. Progestins, on the other hand, can lower the HDL, or good cholesterol, level. What effect will that have on the heart? The PEPI Trial and other studies aim to find out, but results won't be available until late 1994 or early 1995.

What to Discuss with Your Doctor

Whenever your physician prescribes a new medication or renews an old one, it's a good idea to discuss possible side effects. It may help to write your questions down ahead of time so that in the flurry of making it to your doctor's appointment you don't forget what you had meant to ask. A doctor's office is a perfect place to have amnesia!

Once you begin to enter menopause you will probably want to talk with your doctor about ways to deal with this change in your hormone levels. This chapter has presented the pharmacological alternatives. Other chapters will deal with alternative therapies. Dr. Judd, who is cautiously in favor of pharmacological estrogen replacement, suggests that "there are reasons to consider hormones. It is a hard dilemma and it's often an emotional one. However, it's an elective thing—it's not like you're dying of pneumonia and you have to take the penicillin or expire. In this case, you can quietly sit down and think through the pros and cons of its everyday application. What makes some sense to me is that this is prophylactic therapy. We do so much better with prophylactics than we do with treatment of actual conditions [such as osteoporotic hip fractures]. So it's preventative health and that makes it attractive."

In the next chapter I'll talk about what conditions HRT can protect against, and who can benefit most from the therapy.

COMMONLY PRESCRIBED HORMONES

Compound type	Brand name (Manufacturer)	Form/Dosages
estradiol	Estrace (Mead Johnson)	Tablets/1 or 2 mg Cream/0.01%
	Estraderm (Ciba-Geigy)	Patch/0.05 mg/24 hrs. or 0.1 mg/24 hrs.
conjugated estrogens	Premarin (Wyeth-Ayerst)	Tablets/0.3, 0.625, 0.9, 1.25, 2.5 mg Cream/0.0625%
quinestrol	Estrovis (Parke-Davis)	Tablets/0.1 mg
estropipate	Ogen (Abbott)	Tablets/0.625, 1.25, 2.5, 5.0 mg
medroxy-progesterone acetate (progestin)	Provera (Upjohn), Amen (Carnrick)	Tablets/2.5, 5, 10 mg

3

Who Can Benefit from HRT?

. . .

Eva, who's in her mid-60s, started hormone re-
placement therapy at age 59. "My mother was not
definitely diagnosed with osteoporosis, but she
went from being a very statuesque 5'7½" to being
no more than 5 foot 3. In fact, I've lost height
too—I was 5'5½" and I'm now at about 5'4½".
As far as I know, there has been no cancer in my
family. So that piece [of the decision] didn't worry
me. Osteoporosis, on the other hand, was much
more likely. So I was willing to take a gamble, par-
ticularly since I had had some back problems
around the age of 39."

There are many of us who can recall women in the family
who began shrinking as they got older. We may even have
thought of this as inevitable. It may not be, as researchers cited
in this chapter point out.

Eva is in good health and had a compelling family history as reason enough to consider HRT. In this chapter, we'll hear from three other women who came to the decision in slightly different ways. Each story points out how women can benefit from hormone replacement therapy. I'll focus on the reasons that these women and their doctors chose hormone replacement to alleviate current symptoms and to prevent future disease.

"Actually," says Margie, age 63, "I think meno-
pause just kind of sneaked up on me. Twice while I
was sitting down I got warm in the face. After it
was all over I wondered, 'What was that all
about?' and then I remembered, 'Oh, that must be
what they call a hot flash.'

"Probably two years or more after my final
period, my nurse practitioner was unable to get a
perfectly clean reading from my Pap smear. We
went on like that for a couple of years. Finally,
she said, 'I don't see any evidence of cancer, but I
can't in all good conscience let you go on having
less than perfect Pap smears.' So I had my first
D&C [dilatation and curettage—a dilating of the
cervix and scraping of the uterine wall]. That was
perfectly normal as far as cancer was concerned,
but what they found was excess endometrial cells.

"After that, the doctors in the practice felt I
should menstruate again to see if my Paps would
clear up. First I used the estrogen cream and then
took the Premarin and Provera pill. I started hav-
ing periods again, and my Pap smears cleared up

46

right away. They later told me that when I went through menopause, I continued to have a high enough estrogen level so that my body was still producing the thicker endometrial lining, but there was no progesterone there to trigger shedding of the lining. I continued to have periods for quite a few years. I wouldn't have taken it that many years if my doctors hadn't advised it.

"When I changed doctors and got a specialist, he told me he had been a part of the studies, had read the research, and he verified the reports of the benefits. So I have continued hormone replacement therapy. I switched to the patch. And I'm very pleased with the way I feel."

For Mary, now 62, menopause was a different story. She vividly recalls the physiological discomforts: "My brother, who's a physician, thought that I was needlessly uncomfortable because I was having a lot of hot flashes. He'd say, 'Why don't you take estrogen? It's so silly for you to be going through this.'

"I was just not willing to do it. I felt that it was contra-nature and I didn't want to get involved. But subsequent to menopause, I spoke with a cousin of mine who's an internist and for whom I have a high regard. She persuaded me that it was a wise course to take. So I went to a gynecologist and she agreed with everybody else, that HRT had protective benefits against osteoporosis and heart disease. So that was how I began using it. There's

*no history of breast cancer or anything of that sort
in my family.*

*"The gynecologist suggested that it [HRT]
was also going to be good for my hair, skin, and
energy, but as far as those things are concerned, I
really haven't noticed any positive or negative effects of the medication."*

While even its strongest detractors, such as Sidney M.
Wolfe, M.D., Director of Public Citizen's Health Research
Group in Washington, D.C., state that HRT on a short-term
basis can be a good idea to alleviate the symptoms of menopause, it's the long-term use of HRT that stirs the greatest
debate. Private physicians, public health officials, and researchers are now telling women that to get maximum protective effects against osteoporosis and, perhaps, heart disease,
they should remain on the therapy for 10, 15, even 20 years.

Dr. Karen Blanchard, a Santa Monica-based gynecologist, states, "I think as long as you're a woman and you're
alive, you need it. Now, if you're looking only for prevention
of osteoporosis, and it takes between 15 and 20 years for
osteoporosis to develop, you could probably stop it at 85. If
you're looking for its benefit to the cardiovascular system,
well, its benefit goes on for as long as you take it. If you're
looking at its benefit in terms of increased blood flow to the
vagina and to the base of the bladder, so that women are in
more control of their bladder and can enjoy their sexual lives,
then I think it probably should continue as long as women
urinate and have sex. There are lots and lots of benefits to
estrogen, and as long as you want those benefits, then it seems
to me that that's when you take it."

Most women who ask their doctors for hormone replacement therapy want to alleviate symptoms during menopause. However, as we saw with Eva, Margie, and Mary, that's not always the case. For women like Margie, the symptoms of menopause may be no big deal. For those like Mary, it's preferable to tough it out without hormones during menopause, even though they may decide later to take them for other reasons.

Once through the menopause, the most common indication for either continuing the therapy or starting it long-term is to prevent osteoporosis. A family history of heart disease may be another indication. Long-term therapy is also given to women who've had either complete hysterectomies or oophorectomies (to protect the bone and other tissues and organs from estrogen loss), or to premenopausal women who are amenorrheic, as a protection against both endometrial cancer and osteoporosis. There are other less common reasons as well, such as replacing hormone function in women with pituitary problems. But let's look at the more common indications one at a time:

The Bone Question

Bone mass is probably at its peak during a woman's early 20s. At age 35 bone mass begins to decrease in both sexes. So actually, women should pay attention to protecting their bones long before menopause. Health practitioners recommend that you replace calcium at the recommended dosage of 1,000 mg a day at age 30, rather than waiting until later. They also stress the importance of weight-bearing exercise for maintaining skeletal strength. (See Chapter Seven on alternatives to HRT for more tips on calcium replenishment.)

Since osteoporosis is primarily a disease of old age, it can, and does, happen to anyone, male or female. However, women *are* more at risk than men. While men continue to lose a small percentage of bone (3% to 5% per decade) at about the same rate throughout their lives, bone loss for women is accelerated during the first several years after menopause. It is estimated that postmenopausal women lose at least *3% per year.* A woman may lose about 20% of her bone density over and above the normal age-related bone loss during the six years following menopause. "It is ubiquitous in every culture that you tend to lose bone after menopause," says Dr. Robert Lindsay, a reproductive endocrinologist, chief investigator at the Helen Hayes Hospital's Regional Bone Center in New York, and a leading researcher in the treatment of osteoporosis.

Why is this? What scientists now know is that estrogen is key to **bone remodeling,** a process that takes place continuously inside the bone marrow, where large multinuclear cells (called osteoclasts) act on old bone cells and break them down (resorption). Then new bone is formed, and the cycle repeats.

Bone resorption and reformation is a delicately balanced process. Up until your mid-30s there tends to be more reformation of new bone than resorption of old. Then, at about 35, that balance is tipped the opposite way. Resorption begins to outweigh reformation, leading to **osteopenia,** or loss of bone mass. Certain substances, such as caffeine and the chemicals in cigarettes, contribute to increased bone resorption, as does normal aging. Medical conditions such as hyperthyroidism can also speed up bone resorption, because the excess parathyroid hormone stimulates the activity of the osteoclasts.

Senile osteoporosis is another fact of aging. But as stated by Danish chemist Claus Christiansen in Great Britain's *Journal of Steroid Biochemistry and Molecular Biology* (March 1990), "Postmenopausal bone loss is mainly estrogen-dependent." In order for bone remodeling to maintain skeletal integrity, estrogen needs to be present in sufficient levels. Type I, or postmenopausal, osteoporosis, according to Thurman and Marjorie Gillespy, both M.D.s (*Radiologic Clinics of North America*, January, 1991) "is seen in women within 15 to 20 years of the menopause." It's most likely caused, they state, by perimenopausal and postmenopausal estrogen deficiency, which causes increased bone remodeling and subsequent bone loss. Estrogen deficiency also lowers vitamin D levels, which affect calcium absorption, and this may exacerbate bone loss.

"In the past we didn't know that there were estrogen receptors in bone," says Dr. Carolyn Kaplan, reproductive endocrinologist. "Now we do. So we're aware of a direct protective effect of estrogen on bone, in some way. However, we don't know for a fact that taking estrogen will stimulate bone growth." It simply arrests the loss, so that there is less resorption during bone remodeling.

Says Dr. Robert Lindsay of the Helen Hayes Hospital's Regional Bone Center, "There are other types of osteoporosis than those induced by estrogen deficiency. But if you have gotten or you are getting osteoporosis because you have gone through menopause, it will not be prevented by taking calcium alone." In that case, estrogen will be needed to arrest bone loss.

Can you ensure that you won't be at risk for osteoporosis? No, because some of the risk factors (see the next section) are not preventable. Other risk factors, however, are lifestyle-related, and that's why one of the first steps in preventing osteoporosis, says Dr. Lindsay, is to start strengthening the bones *before* menopause. "Having an adequate amount of calcium in your diet is the first thing, because it stops you from robbing the skeleton to keep up the calcium in the blood." The body requires calcium for a variety of processes, such as contraction of muscles, beating of the heart, and clotting of blood. When the level of calcium in the blood drops due to inadequate intake, more calcium is taken from the bones. Dr. Lindsay says, "We advocate that people get an adequate calcium intake from their diet, and if they can't get it from the diet, they ought to take calcium supplements. A small, 200 mg supplement at each meal, coupled with dietary sources, should supply an average of 1,000 mg per day."

The good health habits we practice today *are* a hedge against the development of skeletal problems later in life. Other factors do, however, enter in.

Who's at Risk?

Once she passes through menopause, a woman will spend her remaining years in what doctors call an "estrogen deficient" state. That's neither good nor bad, it's just a fact of life. The ovaries no longer produce estrogen from the androgen precursors, and even though other body tissues are capable of converting precursors to estrogens, it's nowhere near the level that exists during a woman's menstruating years.

While all women may be at risk for estrogen-deprived osteoporosis, there are some women who are considered at higher risk:

- Women with family members who had or have osteoporosis

- Women who are thin and have a frail build. Margie fits this profile: She's always been thin, and she's Caucasian (see below).

- Women who are Caucasian or Asian. Current medical thought is that African-American women are less at risk. "We have a study right now," says Dr. Robert Lindsay, "in which we're looking at why it is that, in their early 20s, black women have slightly higher bone mass than their white counterparts. The presumption is that since they have higher bone mass, it takes them slightly longer to become osteoporotic, but that's never been proved either."

  We don't know the reason for the higher bone mass, although, posits Lindsay, it may be that historically African-American women tended to have to work hard all their lives and therefore had more weight-bearing stress on their bones. Even these data are beginning to change, says Lindsay, with the most recent evidence showing that African-American women are starting to catch up to Asian and Caucasian women in terms of developing osteoporosis.

- Women who smoke cigarettes. If you are a smoker, you are depleting the calcium in your bones. But what if you used to smoke and quit several years ago? Does that lessen your risk from this factor? It's very hard to tell, according to Dr. Carolyn Kaplan. She points out that smoking seems to hasten menopause "because it increases one of the enzymes that breaks down estrogen." The earlier your menopause, the more estrogen-depleted your skeletal system will be.

"I think everyone agrees that if you smoke, you should stop smoking," continues Dr. Kaplan. "We know that if you stop smoking, you will see lung changes reverse over X number of years, but we don't really know that for cardiovascular or osteoporotic disease. We're uncertain of the time frame in which we can say, 'You're now healthier than you were five years ago, or ten years ago.'" At any rate, health professionals agree that quitting smoking is always a good move—for your heart, your lungs, and your bones.

- Women who are sedentary. Over the last decade, mounting data show that **weight-bearing** exercise (in which a load is placed on the skeleton, either through a high- or low-impact aerobics routine, walking, or lifting weights) increases the rate at which bone remodels. You can actually rebuild bone that has decreased in mass by following a regular regimen of weight-bearing exercise (at least 20 minutes three times a week).

- Women whose ovaries were removed before the age of menopause. This might have happened in a complete hysterectomy or an oophorectomy (removal of just the ovaries and not the uterus). Again, if you have been deprived of estrogen before the natural menopause, this sets you up for more bone loss.

- Women who have been compulsive dieters. There's evidence now that radical and rapid shifts in weight can be deleterious not only to your heart, but to your bone. Dr. Lindsay uses the example of ballet dancers, who are bullied by their ballet masters into maintaining sylphlike figures and who therefore resort to poor diets. "Those people are not only calorie-deprived, they're calcium-deprived and they're set up to lose bone," he says. Remember Dr. Lindsay's earlier point that if there isn't sufficient calcium available in your bloodstream, your body will "rob" the skeleton to maintain that proper level.

Consequences of Bone Loss

According to the National Institute on Aging, osteoporosis affects 24 million Americans. As our population ages, the incidence of osteoporosis is increasing. Osteoporosis increases a person's chances of breaking a bone in the event of a fall or other minor accident, but there are other factors that contribute to more fractures in the elderly: changes in the balance mechanism in the ear, unsteadiness leading to falls, overuse of certain medications that cause dizziness, and so on.

Public health officials and medical people are concerned about the costs, personal and economic, of an aging baby boom generation more at risk for serious fractures of the hip and spine. Such fractures require lengthy and costly hospitalizations, subjecting the bedridden patient to the risk of pneumonia, thromboembolism, and death. What physicians are arguing for is a chance to prevent this enormous loss of life and quality of life by prescribing HRT to postmenopausal women *before* there is a serious problem.

Women themselves are in favor of prevention. Margie was an avid reader of Adelle Davis's books on healthy eating and nutrition, and she still takes her vitamin C religiously. She points out, "I believe in sickness prevention. If we're complaining about the high cost of health care for seniors, then we ought to provide them with this [HRT] instead of a $10,000 hip replacement!"

HRT—The Gold Standard for Prevention?

There's no shortage of professional advice about ways to prevent osteoporosis: Get adequate daily calcium, engage in weight-bearing exercise, stop smoking, avoid alcohol and caffeine. But according to Gail A. Greendale, M.D., and her co-authors, writing in the *Journal of General Internal Medicine* (November–December 1990), HRT remains the "gold standard" in osteoporosis prevention. That's because there's no getting around the fact that estrogen is absolutely critical to the process of bone remodeling. It retards the resorption of bone.

Danish and American researchers have demonstrated that HRT (typically .625 mg conjugated estrogens, combined with a progestin for a woman with intact uterus) immediately stabilizes bone loss. In studies done by Lindsay and his colleagues, hormone replacement therapy, combined with total calcium intake (diet and supplements) of 1,500 mg a day, actually produced an increase in both vertebral bone mass and bone mass at the femoral neck (top of the thigh bone). One part of the Framingham Study, published in the *New England*

Journal of Medicine in 1987, stated that HRT reduces the risk of hip fractures by half.

Despite all its good press (or perhaps because of all the *bad* press!), HRT, or CHT (combined hormone therapy), as it's sometimes called, is being used by only about 10% of the postmenopausal women in the United States, according to researcher Howard Judd, now at UCLA. Others put that percentage higher, at about 20%. The most common reason for prescribing the therapy is not prevention of future disease, but ameliorating the symptoms of menopause.

So it's tricky: The physician is trying to urge the patient to consider something that will probably prevent future disease. But there is considerable concern that such long-term use of female hormones will actually trigger more incidence of breast cancer. In addition, hormone replacement therapy doesn't offer the same kinds of tangible results as other therapies. For instance, when you take antibiotics to treat a bacterial infection, you usually feel an improvement within a few days. A woman on HRT may not feel different with the therapy, and usually can't see what it's doing for her bones.

Still, the risk of osteoporosis is real, and Dr. Kaplan and others urge women to schedule regular office visits to talk with their physicians about the pros and cons of HRT. A good time to do that is *before* your menopausal years.

More and more women are experiencing an early menopause, perhaps due to our high-stress lives, so it's not too early to start these discussions in your early to mid-40s. Many women can look to their mothers for clues as to when to expect the onset of menopause. However, the conventional wisdom that women who begin menstruating earlier tend to go through menopause later has not been scientifically validated. The average age of menopause is still 51, but there are measures you can take earlier to lessen your chances of osteoporosis. And there may be ways to screen your bone and predict your future risks. Bone density studies (sophisticated, noninvasive X-rays of the hip and spine) are expensive, but may be worthwhile if you have a family history of the disease. (For more information on bone density studies, see Chapter Nine.)

If you're in the high-risk category for osteoporosis, you and/or your doctor may already be considering HRT as a preventative measure. Before you make a decision, you'll also want to read the chapters on risk and alternative therapies.

The Symptoms of Menopause

As shown in the contrasting experiences of Margie (who had only one or two mild hot flashes) and Mary (who suffered considerable discomfort), menopause is evidenced in radically different ways. I'll list below the range of symptoms that can occur due to the fluctuating hormone levels in your body. Following that, I'll give some examples of how hormone replacement therapy deals with these changes.

Your Periods Change

During your perimenopausal years, you'll begin to notice changes in your cycle. Perhaps your periods will be shorter and the blood flow lighter. You may go for longer periods without menstruating and then have a particularly heavy blood flow. You have more anovulatory cycles, times when an egg is not released from your ovaries. Unless you are undergoing blood tests at the time (which would measure levels of estradiol, FSH, and LH), it may not be possible to tell if you are having an anovulatory cycle, though you might notice it by the *absence* of sensation at a time of the month when you usually ovulate. Many women know when they are ovulating because they can feel a small cramping sensation on either side of the abdomen at the time that the ovary releases an egg.

Usually a woman's periods will gradually become more infrequent, although some women may abruptly stop menstruating altogether. Often when women's periods stop, they initially consult their doctors because they fear they might be pregnant. There is no predicting how your own menopause will happen. Cessation of menses may or may not be accompanied by the additional changes of menopause.

Your Body Changes

There is great change going on inside your body during menopause. Some are quite noticeable to you: your breasts may flatten and thin out and your vaginal walls may thin and get dry (a condition called "vaginal atrophy"). Menopause causes the pH balance in your vagina to change, and this can mean an increased incidence of vaginitis. The drying leads to what doctors call dyspareunia, difficult or painful intercourse.

Your uterus becomes smaller. The muscles in your pelvic floor lose elasticity and strength, and the bladder and lining of the urethra also thin. The result of this can be *very* noticeable—a tendency towards incontinence (a feeling of urgency when urinating), and more bladder infections.

Hot flashes begin to occur—barely eventful for Margie, extremely disruptive for Mary. Some women report waking up drenched in so much sweat that they have to change the sheets. Hot flashes may also contribute to menopausal insomnia. Loss of estrogen, experts believe, may interfere with REM (rapid eye movement) sleep, which is the deepest and most restful phase of the sleep cycle. Hot flashes also occur during the daytime. Nancy, 49, takes off her sweater at least three times a day and fans herself until the hot flash passes.

The other important change, already discussed at length above, is the loss of bone mass due to insufficient quantities of estrogen in the bone remodeling process.

The Mental/Emotional Changes

Historically, menopause was thought to be related to emotional disorders. Scientific thought is now changing on this issue. Women's rights advocates have pointed out that seeing menopause as a "disorder" or hysterical ailment tends to belittle women. Modern medicine concedes that there is no clear-cut cause-and-effect relationship between menopause and depression. Nonetheless, many women do report some very specific neurological effects of menopause, such as a failing memory and mental confusion. Others report feeling more moody. But it's hard to pin emotional instabilities on menopause per se. As some healthcare practitioners note, if a woman's response to stress in the past has been to become depressed, then the extra stresses of the menopause may trigger that response even though they don't cause it.

Also often cited is a loss of libido, or sexual desire. Physicians aren't sure, however, how much of this is due to vaginal atrophy. If intercourse becomes difficult and painful, this naturally has a negative effect on sexual desire. But libido is a complicated mechanism. As endocrinologist Kaplan points out, there are known chemical components for sexual desire. Androgens, or male hormones, are present in your skin, fat, adrenal, and ovarian tissues. Before menopause, your ovaries turn these precursor androgens into estrogens. After menopause, the ovaries continue to make testosterone and other androgens. In women who have had surgical castration, according to Kaplan, hormone replacement with estrogen and progestin will not restore former levels of precursor androgens. For women with surgical menopause who still report loss of libido even after HRT, a small amount of testosterone (an androgen) may be prescribed, and that usually helps.

In our society, menopause is an emotionally charged event. Dr. Cynthia A. Stuenkel, an internist, reproductive endocrinologist, and associate professor of medicine and reproductive medicine at the UCSD School of Medicine, concedes that society's effect on a woman's feelings about aging is a complicated issue. For instance, she points out that in Southern California "the attitudes about aging are more negative than they are in the Northeast, where I think women are much more comfortable with gray hair and wrinkles and the stature that comes with aging. But as for fear of aging altering emotional symptoms, I haven't done any formal studies of this and I haven't really seen it in my patients."

How Estrogen Can Help

"There were nights," recalls Nicky, "when I'd wake up drenched. I'd get up and have to change my nightgown. It didn't happen too much during the day, thank goodness, but some of the evenings were disgusting."

Doctors estimate that 75% to 85% of women experience hot flashes during menopause. For most, these symptoms will subside in about two years. But while they are happening, hot flashes make some women extremely uncomfortable. Most hot flashes occur at night, causing sleep to be severely disrupted. Sleep deprivation can make anyone feel on edge. So if hot flashes are disruptive, estrogen, in either pill, cream, or patch form, will alleviate or cure them altogether.

Estrogen can take care of vaginal atrophy as well. Dryness and thinning of the vagina are reversed on HRT. For women who are sexually active, this is a definite plus. "Penetration becomes painful," Nicky told me. "My doctor told me that as long as I'm having sexual relations, estrogen will keep the vagina moist." This is because estrogen increases blood flow to the vaginal tissues.

Amenorrhea and Early Estrogen Deficiency

Anita, age 40, started hormone replacement therapy a year ago on the advice of her gynecologist. A slender woman, she had been amenorrheic (had not had a period) since the age of 20, and physicians throughout those years had done lots of hormone tests to check her estrogen levels. Although it was usually in the low-to-normal range, her current gynecologist urged Anita to try HRT in order to have periods again. This would restore the protective benefit of estrogen for her bone mass.

"I've been taking the cycle of Premarin and Provera every third month, because my doctor and I were concerned about breast cancer. I'm sort of young to be on HRT. Taking the hormones in this way will be a low dosage, but enough to give me the benefits of estrogen for my bones. I started out having a fairly light period and now I get it rather heavily for about seven days and I get a lot of symptoms—really severe abdominal cramping. My doctor thinks that's a result of the uterus being stimulated after all these years. I also get very bad breast pain and some discharge. I don't feel wonderful on it. This month I'm going to start taking Ogen [manufactured by Abbott, this is synthetic estrogen, estropipate]. If the symptoms lessen with the Ogen, then that'll be okay."

The good news is that at her annual gynecological exam, Anita's doctor said the tissue in her vagina looked "much better, less hormone depleted."

As a result of HRT, Anita will be decreasing her chances of developing bone loss and cardiovascular problems, which I'll discuss next. Often, according to researcher Leon Speroff, amenorrheic women can experience bone loss that is comparable to that of postmenopausal women.

These are the same reasons for prescribing HRT to women who've had their ovaries removed.

Your Heart May Get Protection, Too

The major cause of death in the United States is still heart disease, although cancer is close behind. Until the age of menopause, a woman is protected much more than a man against heart disease and heart attack. After menopause, though, her risk quickly rises to become equal with that of a man.

After much public health education, we are all familiar with the risk factors for heart disease: obesity, excessive consumption of fats, a history of smoking, excessive use of alcohol, family history of heart disease, high blood pressure.

Researchers have found that women taking estrogens experience a good effect on their blood lipid levels, thought to be a major predictor of heart attack. Too much bad cholesterol (LDL) in your blood can cause atherosclerotic deposits on your artery walls, leading to blockage and subsequent heart attack or stroke. On the other hand, higher levels of HDL (good cholesterol) seem to protect against this buildup of plaque. Estrogen raises the levels of HDL in the blood.

So why not just prescribe estrogens for those with high risk factors as a preventative measure? There is some evidence that this might be a good idea. One interesting study was conducted by Brian Henderson, M.D., of the University of Southern California's Comprehensive Cancer Institute. He and several colleagues studied 8,881 women in Leisure World, a retirement community near San Diego, for a period of eight years. There were 1,447 deaths during that period, 94 of which were due to myocardial infarction (heart attack). The researchers found that current users of HRT, who had been on the therapy for the past 15 years, had a 40% reduction in overall mortality, compared with nonusers. In addition, the well-publicized Nurses' Study (*New England Journal of Medicine,* September 12, 1991) found a reduction in heart attack risk among women who used estrogen.

There are a couple of problems with these conclusions, however. Although estrogen raises HDL and lowers LDL, physicians do not prescribe estrogens alone to women who still have an intact uterus. That is because unopposed estrogen can lead to increased risk of endometrial cancer, as discussed earlier. So progestins are added to "oppose" the estrogen, induce menstruation, and protect against endometrial cancer.

But the progestins appear to *lower* HDL levels slightly, thus undermining the protective effect of estrogen on blood lipids.

The current Postmenopausal Estrogen/Progestin Interventions (PEPI) Trial, sponsored by the National Institutes of Health and being conducted at seven major academic institutions across the country, is looking at the dosages of estrogen and progestin to evaluate their effect on blood lipids and other factors. Researchers want to know whether progestin can be given in smaller amounts, perhaps every day, instead of the last 10 days of the monthly cycle, and thus have less effect on lowering HDL. Results won't be known until early 1995, because the test is a double-blind, randomized drug trial. This means that the study subjects, 875 women in all, were randomly assigned to four different combinations of estrogen and progestins. A fifth group was assigned to a placebo. Researchers do not know who is assigned to which group, so they have no way of prejudicing or predicting the outcome of the study.

But there is another wrinkle in the estrogen-cardiovascular controversy. While we think that estrogen may help prevent heart disease, we don't know for sure. And we don't know whether this potentially protective effect is accomplished through the mechanism of raising the HDL level and causing LDL to fall. Howard Judd's view is that estrogens probably do prevent heart disease, but not through an HDL-LDL mechanism. Rather, it may be through "other mechanisms that are directly involved with the blood vessels. But that's a *personal* view," he confesses, "not a proven fact."

But whatever the mechanism, the protection from heart attacks has been proven. This can be a powerful factor in your decision about HRT. The section entitled "Risk Factors for Heart Disease" in Chapter 8 can help you assess your own potential risk.

Conclusion

Aside from the concrete benefits of protection against bone disease, and possibly heart disease, as well as relief from the discomforts of menopause, there is the very real, although less quantifiable, "quality of life" issue. If women are taking estrogens for menopausal symptoms, they experience day-to-day benefits. Vaginal dryness is no longer a problem, and hot flashes are diminished if not eliminated. Their quality of life is measurably improved.

Notes Dr. Kaplan, "In terms of your quality of life, of how you feel on a day-to-day basis, you can eliminate a lot of discomfort—as well as prevent vertebral compression fractures that may lead to back pain and loss of height as a woman gets older."

If quality of life and prevention of bone loss are our primary considerations, the estrogen decision is a fairly clear one. But for those women who have family histories of breast cancer, the choices become more complex. We'll discuss those risks in the next chapter.

CHAPTER

4

Risks of Hormone Replacement Therapy

• • •

"Estrogen is a carcinogen. It causes cancer in animals, and if it were something in the chemical world, it would be banned."
—LEWIS KULLER, Ph.D.,
Epidemiologist, University of Pittsburgh
School of Public Health

"Sure, menopause is a natural event, and sure, taking hormones afterwards is pharmacologic, not physiologic. But it's a judgment you make. I respect the person who says, 'I don't want to take drugs.' Fine, that's a choice you have to make. On the other hand, I would hope my wife would take an appropriate program to keep her alive longer."
—LEON SPEROFF, M.D.,
Reproductive Endocrinologist,
Oregon Health Sciences University

67

*"For most women, the trade-offs for long-term use
[of HRT] aren't worth it."*
—SIDNEY M. WOLFE, M.D.,
Director, Public Citizen Health Research Group

When it comes to long-term estrogen replacement therapy,
everyone disagrees—the experts, practicing physicians,
the drug companies, and consumer groups. There is, however,
something upon which all factions agree: that for certain
women there are definite risks. For instance, if you have a
history of thrombophlebitis, embolism, impaired liver function, sickle cell disease, or abnormal, unexplained vaginal
bleeding (possibly indicating the presence of endometrial cancer), you cannot take estrogens. And as we saw in Chapter
Two, even if you aren't in these highest risk groups, there can
be side effects you should watch out for. Most troublesome is
the relationship between estrogens and breast cancer. The
problem is that the jury's still out on this crucial question.
How, then, are women to make their own individual decisions?

Debbie, a 44-year-old surgical nurse, finds herself in a
quandary about this question right now. Two years ago she was
surprised to find out that she was already perimenopausal.
With an impending early menopause, Debbie's doctor told her
she should start thinking about estrogen replacement therapy.
She's in favor of HRT for its advantages: lessening of menopausal symptoms and protection against osteoporosis and possibly cardiovascular disease.

But there's a problem: Her father's mother had breast
cancer, and Debbie herself has already had a benign tumor

removed from her right breast. Because of her family history, she was dead-set against HRT a year ago. "I was pretty adamant about it then, but now I'm kind of wavering and I'm not sure what to do."

Debbie has done lots of reading—articles in medical journals, items in health and women's magazines, anything she can get her hands on. Because she has a staff position at Touro Infirmary, a large hospital in downtown New Orleans, Debbie is in a position to talk to lots of different doctors. "They [physicians] tell you to get another opinion, but they all have *different* opinions! That isn't any help at all." Right now, she says in exasperation, "I'm just sitting on the fence."

As her estrogen levels fall off, Debbie knows she must make a decision within the next two years and feels pressured to do so. Another worrisome factor is what she thinks may be a trend in surgeries at the hospital. Over the past few years, she has noticed that women coming in for mastectomies seem to be getting younger and younger. "I asked the surgeon if this is because of more diligent screening, or because people are getting breast cancer at a younger age. He told me, 'We're hoping that it's because of more diligent testing.' We're *hoping?* That doesn't make you feel very good!" Debbie's course for now is to "wait and see" and collect as much information as she can.

Many women may be facing the same dilemma when told that HRT is a possibility for them. Here's an example of just how conflicting the information from experts can be:

I questioned Dr. Howard Judd, a UCLA reproductive endocrinologist and principal investigator in the NIH multi-center PEPI Trial, about the safety of HRT for a woman with a history of breast cancer on her father's side of the family. He replied, "To me, that's an easy one, because a paternal grandmother is a second-degree relative. That's a distant relative in regard to breast cancer. It's primary relatives—your mother or sisters—that are of more concern than your grandmothers. So the chance of breast cancer risk in that individual is only minimally increased over a woman of average risk."

Added reproductive endocrinologist Carolyn Kaplan, an M.D. in a Santa Monica group practice, having a paternal grandmother with breast cancer is the same risk as having a maternal grandmother with breast cancer.

Even though Judd believes the risk for breast cancer in a woman with second-degree family history of the disease is not as great, he nevertheless offers cautions. A woman with a relatively remote family history of cancer, he says, "should not believe that if she chooses not to take estrogen she cannot get breast cancer. Neither should she believe that if she does take estrogen she *will* get breast cancer. Your chances [as a woman] of having breast cancer are a hundred times what my chances are. Part of that increased risk is that you've been exposed to far more estrogen than I have."

There's the rub. Just by being a woman, your exposure to estrogen is much higher than a man's. Remember the balance of power we talked about in Chapter One? Both sexes produce male and female hormones, but it's the prevalence of one or the other that gives us our secondary sex characteristics. Estrogen causes a woman's breasts to develop. And it causes breast cancer to develop. Some men, in fact, do develop breast cancer, although it is rare. In order to sort out the relative risks of long-term estrogen replacement therapy, it's helpful to understand the link between sex hormones and breast cancer.

Do Estrogen and Breast Cancer Go Hand in Hand?

I had my first brush with the fear of breast cancer when I was 20. While away at college, I found a lump in my left breast. After a mammogram and two physical exams, and an unsuccessful attempt to aspirate (suction fluids from) the lump, my family doctor decided to operate. I remember coming out of anesthesia, putting my hand on my bandaged left breast, and asking the recovery room nurse, "Is it still there?" After she nodded, I was able to go back to sleep. The lump had been a benign fibroadenoma, a finding that made the bruising and pain after the operation easier to take.

Later, doctors told me I had fibrocystic disease, a benign condition of the breasts in which clumps of tissue occasionally produce noncancerous lumps. However, there are many types of fibrous cysts in the breasts, and only a few exhibit precancerous atypical hyperplasia (abnormal overgrowth of cells) or calcifications that go on to become cancer. Interestingly, some doctors now argue that this "disease" should be called fibrocystic "condition," to take it out of the realm of fear for women.

According to Dr. Leon Speroff, a top researcher at Oregon Health Sciences University, the two main reasons that women stop taking estrogen therapy are monthly bleeding and the fear of cancer. Indeed, it's the fear of cancer that stops many women from even asking their doctors about estrogens in the first place.

Not only does breast cancer threaten your life, it can temporarily, even permanently, wreak havoc with your sexual

71

identity. Even with a strong family support system, the disfigurement of radical mastectomy and the agony of treatment can be especially hard to bear.

When Growth Leads to Cancer

Why is it that cancer attacks the very organs that define you as a woman? As you may recall from Chapter One, "Estrogen's Role in Your Health," estrogens are sex steroids—they're growth hormones. They send a message to estrogen-receptive tissues (breasts, skin, and bone), telling them to grow and proliferate. The cells in your uterine lining are "told" to grow, because that's the way your body prepares itself to receive a fertilized ovum for implantation. When those cells proliferate without being shed, the potential for cancer arises. During a woman's reproductive years, the body has a natural way of protecting against this condition: Every month that you aren't pregnant, the extra cells are shed during your menstrual period.

The rise of endometrial cancer in the early and mid-1970s, mostly as a result of higher-dose estrogens (for oral contraception and for postmenopausal replacement), was addressed by adding progestins, which act as anti-proliferatives for the endometrial lining. Although this diminishes most of the risk of uterine cancer, there's now concern that progestins may also stimulate tumor growth in the breasts. Study results on this point, once again, are conflicting. Some researchers intimate that adding progestins to hormone replacement may *protect* you from getting breast cancer!

Estrogen binds to receptors inside cell nuclei, stimulating those cells to grow. At some point, the growth can go awry and the cells can multiply and form malignant masses. So there's really no great mystery about the connection between estrogen and development of breast cancer. That potential exists in every woman. What *is* unknown, though, is why one woman gets breast cancer while another does not.

Length of Exposure

The occurrence of breast cancer in the United States is increasing at an alarming rate. In 1961, the risk of breast cancer for American women was one in twenty; in the 1970s that increased to one in twelve; now public health officials are putting the risk at one in *nine*.

In addition, researchers and doctors now know more about specific risk factors for breast cancer. These risk factors relate mostly to the length of time that you're exposed to estrogen over your lifetime. Here are the factors taken into consideration to determine increased risk:

- *Age at menarche* (MEN-ark-ee): Did you start menstruating earlier or later than your peers? If you began having periods at nine, as opposed to thirteen, that's four additional years of estrogen exposure, and you're considered more at risk.

- *Age at menopause:* The same rule applies here—if you have an early menopause, then that's fewer years with full-strength levels of estrogen in your system. (But if you experience a very early menopause—the early 40s—this also can set you up for estrogen-deficient changes in bone and cholesterol levels.)

- *Age at primiparity* (first full-term pregnancy): Did you have children before age 30? Pregnancy interrupts the levels of estrogen, and if you have children in your 20s as opposed to having them at age 30 or beyond, you've had a break in those hormones earlier. A woman who has children later has had more of an uninterrupted "dose" of estrogens in her body.

- *Nulliparous* (never having borne a child): If you have never been pregnant, then you've never had a "break" from estrogens.

- *Family history of breast cancer:* A history of breast cancer on either your mother's or father's side of the family can be critical. However, it's more difficult to ascertain how a father's genetics affect a daughter's risk.

- *Other possible factors:*

A HISTORY OF BENIGN BREAST DISEASE: Studies have not borne out an absolute cause-and-effect relationship here. In addition, there are several types of benign breast disease grouped under this umbrella heading, so unless a lumpectomy or aspiration of a lump showed the presence of **hyperplasia** (abnormal cell growth), you are probably not at increased risk.

BREASTFEEDING: Some studies indicate that breastfeeding may offer a protective effect if you breastfeed each infant for at least a year. However, the effect is less marked if your pregnancies occur after age 30.

OBESITY: Women who are more than 20% overweight usually have higher estrogen levels than their thinner counterparts. Their fatty tissues have androgens that can be converted

74

into estrone, one of the body's three estrogen compounds. As a result, these women are generally less estrogen-deficient at the time of menopause, and consequently usually less symptomatic. Since they have more **endogenous** estrogen (originating within the body), they are exposed to more estrogen overall.

While it is helpful to educate yourself about potential risk factors in your health profile, it's not wise to rely on your "score" to predict a disease-free future. Radiologist Gloria Frankl, M.D., of Kaiser Permanente's Sunset Center in Los Angeles, has been head of mammography for 20 years. During that time, her department has conducted more than 40,000 breast X-rays and she's watched the rate of breast cancer increase. She reports that *34% of women whose mammogram showed the presence of a malignant growth had no risk factors whatsoever.* She cautions that the best advice is to follow guidelines about baseline and regular followup mammograms to effectively screen for early disease. (Chapter Nine offers some pointers about commonsense monitoring for all women.)

Now you understand what the body's own manufacture of estrogens can do *prior* to menopause. So what effect does it have on your body to take doses of estrogens *after* menopause?

Studies—What Do They Show? What Do They Know?

After you look at the above risk factors, you might, quite logically, conclude that taking **exogenous** estrogens (developed outside the body, either synthetically or biologically) after menopause quite simply extends the body's exposure to the hormone, compounding risk. Not so, according to a variety of experts.

The question of potential breast cancer risk with long-term HRT is "very difficult," says Dr. Karen Blanchard. "There are very good studies that show there is no increased risk of breast cancer, and there are studies that show that there *is* an increased risk. Well, we live in a society where one out of nine women get breast cancer. *Every* woman is at increased risk of breast cancer in our society. However, I don't think the entire picture has been developed, and we'll probably need another generation before that can be answered in an intelligent way."

"What about breast cancer?" asks Dr. Lewis Kuller. "Well, that's the big IF. We don't really completely understand the possible interrelationships. In the past, most women who got estrogen therapy were given it because they were symptomatic during the postmenopausal period. And those women, by definition, are deficient in estrogen, so they are probably at lower risk of cancer, if estrogens are related to cancer.

"Unfortunately," continues Kuller, "the NIH [National Institutes of Health], which should have done these trials 15 years ago, is just now in the process of embarking on such trials. And that's the tragedy of this whole thing. . . . The problem is that right now women just have to look on a piece of paper with a doctor and bet whether they're in group A [at risk for osteoporosis], group B [at risk for heart disease], or group C [at risk for breast cancer] and it's betting based on really shoddy information."

Medical research on the possible link between estrogens and breast cancer is inconclusive for several reasons: 1) scientists haven't been following women who take or have taken

Search Request: K=MENOPAUSE
BOOK - Record 14 of 29 Entries Found

Author: Henkel, Gretchen.

Title: Making the estrogen decision / Gretchen Henkel.

Published: Los Angeles : Lowell House ; Chicago : Contemporary Books,
             c1992.

LOCATION: CALL NUMBER: STATUS:
rockville circulating RG186 .H46 1992   Not checked out
collection

--- Page 1 of 1 -----------

sta: Start over   lo: Long view   n: Next record
h: Help   i: Index   p: Previous record
o: Other options

NEXT COMMAND:

estrogen for long enough periods of time; 2) many studies have been observational, as opposed to controlled, double-blind studies; and 3) not all studies to date are measuring the same factors (dosages, age of women, similar histories, and so forth). Many studies that get attention in this country have been done in Sweden and England, which have different populations from the U.S. In addition, no studies have given HRT to women selected randomly from the population, to see what percentage do or do not develop any cancers. Because study methods vary, it's a little like comparing apples and oranges. For instance, a 1989 Swedish study, which found a 30% increased risk of breast cancer in women who took estrogens, stole headlines the week it was released in the *New England Journal of Medicine,* one of the country's most reputable peer-review medical journals. The form of estrogen used, estradiol, is a synthetic compound that is used in micronized form in the United States (brand name, Estrace). But the Swedish study used higher doses of the estradiol than are prescribed here.

And there's another issue: How do scientists factor in a woman's lifetime exposure to estrogen during her reproductive years, and separate out risk from her own estrogens as opposed to pharmacologic estrogens taken after menopause? That's one of the questions that we have yet to address, notes Dr. Carolyn Kaplan: "It's very difficult to show an effect [of taking estrogen] because you're not talking about giving estrogen to someone who's never had it."

Types of Studies

Medical studies fall into two general categories: experimental and non-experimental. In basic research, experiments are often

77

performed on animals. This is the kind of data that furthers our understanding of physiology and disease processes, but usually doesn't have direct clinical applications. Research projects using people, called clinical trials, supply hard facts about the safety and effectiveness of a particular drug or treatment. For instance, the much-touted PEPI Trial is a controlled, randomized, double-blind drug trial. This means that neither study participants nor researchers know who is being given what form of the medication. The 875 women enrolled in the study are being given either one of four possible combinations of estrogen-progestin, or a placebo. Blood levels of hormone and of cholesterol and clotting factors are measured and tabulated. The results of the study will be published in about two years.

Observational studies fall into the non-experimental category. These studies are usually conducted by epidemiologists, scientists who do research on a group of people (called a cohort) who are free of a particular disease (in this case, breast cancer) and who have varying degrees of exposure to risk factors. The cohort, or group, is followed for a particular time period to allow epidemiologists to determine the incidence rates of the disease in the exposed versus the nonexposed groups. Epidemiologists collect their data from hospitals, national registries kept by the Centers for Disease Control, and insurance company records. Their studies can be prospective (following a cohort into the future) or retrospective (historical or case-control). Retrospective studies start with a group of individuals who have already been diagnosed as having a disease (cases) and compare them with a group of people who do not have that disease (controls) to determine any differences regarding their exposure to possible risk factors.

Medical scientists often complain that the methods of observational studies are not fine enough, and that they are therefore not "good quality" studies. There can be "threats to validity," or biases, inherent in the study design. For instance, the way cases and controls are selected can introduce bias. Several researchers have already noted that women recruited for estrogen studies tend to be white, upper-middle-class women who generally take good care of themselves and are likely to exercise and visit the doctor more frequently. Another complaint about retrospective studies is that they may rely on self-reporting by study participants, whose memories of possible past exposure to potential carcinogens could be faulty. And only relative risk, not true incidence of getting the disease, can be measured.

In prospective studies, especially those in which women using estrogens have had a slightly increased incidence of malignancies show up on mammmograms, scientists argue that there can be a surveillance bias. In other words, because these women were in a study, they were being monitored more closely than the general population, and thus more cases of malignancy were found earlier. You'll read a little bit more about how doctors compare results from various studies in the next section.

Value of Meta-Analyses

Medical science has a valuable tool for looking at the combined results of disparate studies. Conducting a so-called "meta-analysis," scientists take data from various studies, rate the study methods according to the quality of the study, and then draw conclusions based on a statistical analysis. One such study that is currently relied upon by doctors and epidemiologists was published in the April 17, 1991 issue of the *Journal of the American Medical Association*. In the studies judged by three separate reviewers to be of good quality, there was a 30% increased risk of breast cancer if a woman had used non-contraceptive estrogens for 15 years. If that use were extended to 25 years, women could be at 50% increased risk of breast cancer over those who were not taking estrogens. This sounds quite alarming, especially since doctors may advise women to take estrogens for 20 years or longer to protect against bone loss after menopause.

Yet another meta-analysis conducted by a preventive medicine specialist and a pathologist from Vanderbilt University School of Medicine in Nashville was published in the January 1991 *Archives of Internal Medicine*. Drs. Dupont and Page tested the hypothesis that breast cancer risk varies with type and dosage of the estrogen given. They concluded that given the different indications for HRT in premenopausal women (hysterectomies, endocrine disease) and postmenopausal women, the relative risk of breast cancer is directly related to dosage. Thus, women given a higher dosage of estrogens to compensate for loss of their ovaries may be at higher risk of breast cancer, while women given menopausal therapy of .625 mg or less of conjugated estrogens will not have an increased risk. These authors also concluded that this low dosage of conjugated estrogens is not contraindicated in women with a history of benign breast disease. Two meta-analyses, two different conclusions. Where does that leave you?

How to Read a Medical Study

"Study proves that bowling causes cancer—details on the four o'clock news."

Consumers are virtually bombarded with headlines about recent studies these days. Often the net effect of such reporting is that we can add one more item to our list of worries. And in this era of "sound bite" news reports, we may not always get the whole picture, such as, Did the people who bowled also smoke cigarettes? What were their ages? Economic backgrounds? Were their diets poor? When the study is conducted two years later and yields conflicting results, it may not be reported as diligently. Does this mean you should ignore news reports? Of course not. But you may have to do some delving of your own to see whether the study really relates to you personally.

Later in the chapter, you'll hear about one woman who decided to tackle the studies herself. This is time-consuming but not impossible. Public libraries keep indexes of most consumer magazines and newspapers so that you can look for articles written on the subject of estrogens and risk factors. Most major university medical schools have libraries with excellent data bases, and librarians who can assist you in doing a search of relevant studies. If you have a modem connected to your home computer, you can subscribe to various commercial or library data bases for a yearly hookup fee and be charged by the hour while you conduct a data base search. Once you've located promising article titles, you can use the same data base's subscriber service to get copies, or you can go to the medical library and make photocopies yourself.

You'll have to wade through lots of technical jargon, but generally the abstract—a short summary paragraph introducing the published study—offers a good synopsis of the study's findings.

Initial studies of new drug treatments are performed with small numbers of patients. If found to be successful, the drugs will then be given to a larger study population. What you will be looking for when you read such studies, or abstracts of them, is how relevant this study is to *you*. Try to determine:

- Is sample size representative and large enough? For instance, a study done in England on five women taking only estrogen (without progestin) would probably not be relevant to an American Latina considering HRT. Cultural background and diet are extremely different.

- Are types of drugs and dosages similar to what you would be taking? Unless a woman has no uterus, estrogen is almost never given alone in this country. Some earlier studies done in other countries have given estrogens unopposed, or have given different derivatives of the drug than we do in the United States.

- What are the particulars of study participants? If the study determined an increased incidence of breast cancer after estrogen use, what *kind* of breast cancer was it? Did the patients have any other predisposing risks for breast cancer? Keep in mind that researchers may not have taken into account all possible variables.

You may want to photocopy the articles you think are particularly relevant to you, and show them to your doctor.

This can be accomplished in a non-threatening way by asking your physician whether he or she has heard of the study that you believe may be important in your case. Your aim should be to become a better partner with your doctor.

The Decision's Still Yours

All reasonable physicians would agree with Dr. Lewis Kuller when he states that the decision about estrogen therapy should be based on an individualized approach, with the woman and her physician making as rational a decision as possible. That means that you need as much information as possible about your personal risk-benefit ratio.

Listening to the Experts

Dr. Saar Porrath, a radiologist and head of the Women's Breast Center in Santa Monica, points out that all breast cancers are estrogen-dependent—it's just a matter of degree. Still, his opinion is that most women *can* take estrogen therapy because of its benefits. "And," he points out, "there's a big difference between getting breast cancer and dying from it."

I think most women would rather not knowingly increase their chances of even *getting* the disease. On the other hand, Dr. Trudy Bush, an associate professor of epidemiology and gynecology at Johns Hopkins University School of Medicine, has published rather dramatic data comparing new cases and deaths from heart attack with new cases and deaths from breast and uterine cancer. Represented in bar graph form, the data reveal that a woman is three times more likely to get or die from heart disease than breast cancer; and six times more likely to die of coronary disease than breast cancer; and *twelve times* more likely to die of heart disease than uterine cancer.

A physician who sees a patient at risk for osteoporosis is likely to give quite a bit of weight to the issue of quality of life for that woman. Afflicting over 25 million Americans, osteoporosis affects more than half of all women over the age of 65. Someone who develops osteoporosis has a severely restricted life. When the bones are exceedingly thin and porous, even a sneeze can trigger a spinal fracture. That, in turn, can lead to a constellation of other problems—back pain, bladder and kidney discomfort, and more.

But, counters epidemiologist Kuller, we haven't yet seen data from long-term use of postmenopausal estrogens. The average incidence of breast cancer is about four per thousand. (Relative risk of getting cancer is figured *over a lifetime,* while average incidence is figured in the population at present.) If that were doubled, as Kuller thinks it could with large-scale prescription of estrogens, that would be 8% to 10% of postmenopausal women—1.6 million, approximately, who might be getting breast cancer. "That's certainly a quality-of-life issue of substantial importance, too," Kuller points out, because having the disease and going through treatment greatly affect a woman's life.

Who Should Avoid HRT?

Besides those with prior histories of embolisms, liver disease, and other risk factors, there are some women who, given the lack of hard, long-term data, would be wise to avoid postmenopausal estrogen therapy.

For instance, consider the heavy woman who generally will have a higher estrogen level: She is much less likely to

suffer a fracture, according to Dr. Kuller. She also will probably not get as symptomatic during menopause, because she
won't be as estrogen deficient. And she will probably be at
increased risk of breast cancer. "So in my view," says Kuller,
"overweight women, especially with a family history of breast
cancer and especially if they have minimal menopausal symptoms, are a no-no for estrogen therapy right now."

"Now, those heavier women also have a somewhat higher
risk of heart disease. So it presents an interesting problem,
because the estrogens might be very good for them in terms of
heart disease reduction and risk. But I think their risk of getting
breast cancer cancels out the advisability of taking estrogens
to protect against heart disease. They might do better to try
other sorts of treatments."

Listening to Yourself

Given the plethora of conflicting study results, you may begin
to feel overwhelmed by the information and be unsure, just as
Debbie is, of which path to take. You and your doctor are the
final arbiters on this question. One Los Angeles internist told
me about a patient of his who insisted on researching the breast
cancer risk herself. After an early menopause and with a family
history of osteoporosis, this professional woman had taken
HRT for 20 years. However, after she was successfully treated
for breast cancer, her physician advised her he could no longer
prescribe estrogens for her. The patient rejected the physician's
analysis and undertook her own research project. She consulted a renowned oncologist, had him do a journal search, and
on the basis of there being no positive or conclusive correlation
between estrogens and breast cancer, decided to continue with
the therapy.

Dr. Carolyn Kaplan advises women to take charge by doing other kinds of self-care. For instance, every woman should make sure she does a monthly BSE (breast self-examination). Whether you're on HRT or not, this is a valuable tool. And it's just as important for younger women. Dr. Porrath notes that breast cancer in menstruating women seems to be on the increase, confirming what Debbie in New Orleans has also noticed.

One women's clinic I visited after my breast biopsy taught me to keep a sketch of the masses I found in my breasts, and to track them. Knowing the location and approximate size of the lumpy areas allowed me to compare them each month, and to see whether there had been any changes. I key my annual mammogram to my birthday, because it's easier to remember and it's a way of taking care of myself at that time. (Chapter Nine discusses additional self-care monitoring and Chapter Eight offers some guides to help you assess your own benefit-risk profile.)

"The main concern," according to Dr. Kuller, is for people to realize that estrogen is "a drug. It's a drug that causes cancer, it's a drug that has benefits. And we have a very big gray area, in which we don't really know, in spite of what people say, how much of a risk it is in regard to breast cancer—we just do not know that right now."

However, there are alternatives to the benefits of estrogen, maintains Kuller. "For example, a woman can do a lot of things to prevent getting a heart attack. If she knows her lipid levels, she can lower them. If her HDL is too low, she can exercise a little bit to help raise it. If she smokes, she can stop smoking. If she's hypertensive, she can get treated. She can go on a diet and lower her blood pressure. If a diet doesn't work and her lipids are still too high, we have a whole bunch of drugs right now that are much more potent than estrogen in lowering the lipid level."

On the other hand, there are women who can definitely benefit from estrogen therapy, among them women who've had hysterectomies, an early menopause, or severe symptoms while going through menopause. It's important, notes Kuller, not to write off estrogen therapy. "It's ridiculous to write off hormone therapy and say it's dangerous. *Everything* is dangerous.

"People are surprised to find out that anything you do has certain risks. If it's a therapeutic intervention, it carries a risk. The risk can be very small, but still, that person in the numerator [the small fraction at risk] could be you."

Exactly. Looking at Dr. Bush's data, and seeing how relatively small the risk of breast cancer is compared to those of heart disease and osteoporosis, you're tempted to say, Let's go for it. But all those statistics go out the window if you become one of the minority of women who could get breast cancer from this therapy. However, this is also one of those life decisions that you do *not* have to rush. You can start talking to your doctor before you're menopausal. As you'll see in later chapters, there's a lot you can do to prepare yourself.

5.

The Physical Side Effects of HRT—What to Expect and How to Minimize Them

• • •

"I've been taking estrogen for five years and haven't noticed any physical side effects. In fact, this year I've felt better than ever."
            —WENDY, age 40

"I've had all kinds of problems with HRT. First of all, I was bleeding all the time. I went in to see my doctor, and she took me off the hormones. Then I got a bladder infection. At this point I

*don't know what's going on and I'm very an-
noyed. I'm beginning to wonder if I'd simply be
better off without it."*

—NICKY, mid-60s

In this chapter you'll meet several women who've been
taking hormones for varying lengths of time and whose
experiences have been quite different. You'll also meet another two women whose therapy started within the past year,
and whose struggles with side effects have prompted their
physicians to undertake different approaches. Later in the
chapter, you'll get some tips on what to do to deal with side
effects.

What's Normal with HRT?

Wendy, now 40 and the mother of two girls, 9 and 5, had a
complete hysterectomy five years ago, following a severe
ovarian infection. (Her condition was so rare that her physicians were never able to establish a definitive diagnosis.)
Despite having both her ovaries and her uterus removed,
Wendy was at first prescribed a cyclic dose of Premarin and
Provera. "It was hard to adjust," she recalls. "I went through
cycles and got moody, almost like PMS. I felt depressed and I
cried a lot. Of course the other factors were that I'd just had
Nickie (her second child was only three months old at the
time), had gone through surgery, and was separated from my
husband. So I had a lot of things to actually be depressed about.

"After two years, I was switched to a lower dose of estrogen and they took me off the progestin. Now I just take estrogen all the time. And I would say that I feel fabulous. I don't notice any side effects, and I feel as energetic as I've ever felt."

How should you expect to feel when you're on HRT? Wendy and some of the older women I talked with reported no side effects at all. Those with intact uteruses who take a monthly dose of Provera still had menstrual periods, but otherwise experienced no ill effects. For other women, having menstrual periods again is no picnic.

"Am I going to be 90 years old and still having my period? Give me a break!" That's Sophia talking, who is 57 and has a period twice a month on HRT. (Part of her story also appeared in Chapter One.) Her gynecologist prescribed HRT because a hip X-ray, taken 15 years after she went through menopause, revealed that she already had osteoporosis. Her menopause had been an early one. Sophia agreed that HRT was a good idea to combat any further bone loss, but she isn't so sure she likes what's happening to her body. "I never know when I'm going to start my period. It used to be that I could tell because my breasts got sore a few days before. Now my breasts are so sore all the time that I never pay attention, and my period is every 15 days." When I told Sophia that other women also have periods on HRT, she was surprised. "Oh, that's good. I thought I was the only one."

Even though periods are a normal part of HRT (when sequential doses of estrogen and progestin are administered), Sophia has plans to see her physician for a checkup, since her periods occur so close together. The progestin is given expressly for the purpose of triggering menstruation because of its protective effects on the uterus. It's important to understand the *normal* physical effects of taking HRT, as opposed to side effects that *aren't* normal. That way, you'll be able to track your symptoms and notify your doctor of changes.

On the plus side, Sophia's been grateful that her hot flashes have ceased since beginning the HRT. What the therapy is doing for her bones remains to be seen, and she anticipates a follow-up X-ray of them at her yearly checkup.

Sensations like wavelengths traveling through her body troubled Sophia before she started HRT and disappeared after her first few months on the therapy. Now the sensations are back. She mentioned this fact to her physician, who has said they may double the dose of Premarin to see if the uncomfortable feelings go away again.

As we discussed in Chapter Two, there is a normal range of probable side effects of HRT. With both the generic and brand-name forms of the medications, you'll receive a list [in tiny print] of all possible side effects from the drug's manufacturer. (If you're a member of an HMO, you may not get this sheet, but you can ask your pharmacist for printed information.) Ideally such information should also come from your doctor, but this may not always happen. Although the practice of medicine is changing and physicians are becoming increasingly aware of their obligation to patients, there are still those who are too rushed or too cavalier about a woman's symptoms to fully discuss with her all the possible side effects and consequences of this therapy. For instance, Wendy was aware of her need for estrogen after a hysterectomy, and *she* was the one who had to bring up the subject with her doctor.

"I spoke to my gynecologist the day I was going home from the hospital and I was the one who asked, 'Am I going to take estrogen? What's going on? Am I going to turn into an old wreck?' He casually replied, 'Oh yeah, we'll give you a prescription.'"

Wendy's experience was in a clinic setting at a university hospital. Clinicians are often rushed, and there may be so many patients that none of them receives enough time with the doctor.

But even in that kind of situation, it is possible to have a conversation about your prognosis with your physician. You can take a list of questions with you so you don't waste time trying to remember on the spot the specifics about drug side effects or other physical complaints that you want to discuss. If you think you aren't getting the proper attention and care, you can ask to switch doctors. This is *your* right as a patient.

Side Effects—Common to Uncommon

Reading through the list of possible side effects of estrogens can be eye-opening. Many of the body's major systems are affected by estrogen. Of course, some of those effects are the very reason why you may be considering HRT. Other effects may be unwanted and downright dangerous if they're not recognized by you or your doctor.

You already know that your vascular system, your skeletal system, your sexual organs, and your nervous system are affected by estrogens.

The common side effects (sometimes described as "natural, expected and unavoidable"), include:

- fluid retention and weight gain (usually about five pounds)

- stomach upset
- "breakthrough" bleeding (between menstrual periods)
- increased susceptibility to genital yeast infections
- swelling and tenderness of the breasts
- increased vaginal secretions.

Possible adverse effects include:

- allergic reactions of the skin, such as hives, itching, and skin rashes
- headaches
- increased irritability
- increased facial pigmentation.

Serious side effects that warrant attention right away include:

- rise in blood pressure
- depression
- sudden impairment of vision, possibly caused by retinal thrombosis—a blood clot in the eye vessels.

In susceptible individuals, estrogens can also exacerbate thrombophlebitis and lead to stroke or pulmonary embolism, even heart attack. *If you have any history of thrombophlebitis, estrogens are not for you.* This is the most common contraindication for taking estrogens and one that all physicians take into account before prescribing estrogens. But there are other rarer side effects which your physician may not know about or discuss with you. For instance, occasionally estrogens can affect your ability to wear contact lenses; they act on the cornea, changing its curvature so that the lenses are quite uncomfortable.

Check It Out

If you notice the sudden onset of any symptom after beginning HRT, you should report it to your doctor. Depending upon your symptom, he or she may order blood tests, do an endometrial biopsy (in the event of unexplained uterine bleeding), or simply raise or lower the dosage of estrogen and/or progestins to see if that alleviates the symptom. Nicky complains that she had to nudge her doctor a bit about her uncomfortable periods with heavy cramping. But her heavy bleeding had her worried, and now, at least, her doctor is changing her prescription to see if a new form of estrogen will work better for her.

In addition, since estrogens are such potent hormones, a checkup every six months is a good idea. It should include a Pap smear, a breast and pelvic exam, as well as the appropriate blood tests to monitor blood lipid levels. Remember, with the right kind of monitoring, even if there's a problem, you will gather information that will allow you and your doctor to take action. Having real information also helps you to feel more empowered about your own health. Within reason, tracking the critical levels (blood pressure, fats in the blood, Pap smear results) can help you feel in charge of your own body. But beware; sometimes you can become a numbers junkie, fixating so much on the "levels" that you lose perspective. (In Chapter

Nine I give some more tips on commonsense monitoring, knowing what the numbers mean, and doing something about them.)

Should You Discontinue?

When I first met with Nicky, a slender woman in her early 60s, she had been taking hormone replacement therapy for the past seven years. At that time she told me, "If you think I have any answers, you're mistaken. I mean I honestly don't know. I read a lot and consider myself at least halfway intelligent. But even if you try, how completely informed can you ever be on this subject?

"I've had problems. I couldn't use the patch—I was allergic to that. So I went to the pills, taking the estrogen in a daily dosage. I just didn't feel right with that. The doctor asked me *what* didn't feel right, but I couldn't explain it. And another thing, I would love to eliminate having a period, which seems peculiar at my age.

"I'm now taking Estrovis [a lower dosage, .1 mg, of quinestrol, a synthetic estrogen] every ten days and progestin [Provera] the first seven days of the month. I just had a period, and on Tuesday night I had such severe cramps that I had to get up and take an aspirin in the middle of the night."

At that time, Nicky was considering discontinuing HRT, although she wanted the other benefits—protection against osteoporosis ("which, they tell me, is a horror") and possibly heart disease. Still, she wasn't comfortable with the way it was going.

"I'm not a pill-taker, first of all," she explained, "and I don't think doctors are God. I have complications with my breasts that concern me too, but I spoke to the radiologist when I went for my yearly mammogram and he doesn't think that [HRT] is a serious risk. He also thinks I should stay on the pills."

Nicky conceded that everything in her life seemed topsy-turvy since her husband's sudden heart attack and emergency quintuple bypass last spring. She acknowledged that perhaps she was over-worried about the hormone therapy. But the side effects she was experiencing from HRT are troubling. After the heavy bleeding and intense cramping of her last period, she called her gynecologist, who suggested that she keep a diary of her symptoms so that the two of them can track what's happening. I called her the next month and got the story that appears at the beginning of this chapter. Things had gone from bad to worse for her, and she was completely off the hormones, waiting to see if her doctor would advise a D&C to diagnose the cause of her almost continuous bleeding.

As it turned out, her bleeding did not stop when Nicky stopped taking the hormones. After two weeks of this, her physician had her come into the office for an endometrial biopsy. For Nicky this was an uncomfortable procedure, which produced cramping, pain, and fatigue. However, her bleeding receded quickly afterwards. During the course of the biopsy, the physician noticed that her vaginal tissues were getting drier again. She concluded that Nicky wasn't getting *enough* estrogen, as opposed to too much. The imbalance of estrogen to progestin had caused the excess bleeding. She'll be taking a 1 mg dose of Estrace, a synthetic estradiol (days 1 through 25), and 2.5 mg of Provera (days 16 to 25) for the next month to see how it goes. "By now I don't know what I'm doing," Nicky wryly says, referring to her new pill-taking schedule. "This is a very involved, very complex business, and I think doctors are staggering around a little in the dark too." At least Nicky's doctor is responding to her symptoms and trying to find out what will work. Some women have physicians who respond that they will only prescribe textbook dosages and medications. Their patients often just stop taking the medication because it makes them too uncomfortable and their doctors refuse to acknowledge their complaints.

One of the scariest side effects of HRT is abnormal bleeding. A menstrual period is expected, but if you bleed intermittently or profusely, it warrants a much closer look. In Nicky's case, her physician first asked her to monitor her heavy periods. When they didn't subside, she performed an endometrial biopsy (taking a sample of uterine tissue in the office) to be sure that there were no malignancies in the uterus and that the estrogen was not causing such a condition to occur. Some physicians might first try what is called a progesterone challenge test, giving just progestin for a few days to see if that triggers more bleeding. If it does, it can indicate that the endometrial cells are proliferating rapidly. Or it can mean that there is insufficient estrogen to counteract the progesterone. A D&C (dilating of the cervix and scraping of the uterine lining) might be performed if the physician has additional concerns about the uterus. That procedure is usually done in a hospital setting.

Certain women may be more susceptible to the changes that estrogen produces. If you are one of the few women who, for instance, cannot take estrogen because of breast pain, and for whom lowering the dosage does nothing to alleviate that symptom, you may want to discuss the pros and cons of continuing HRT with your doctor.

Likewise, there are some women who tend toward high blood pressure and whose condition might worsen with HRT.

Again, if you're having six-month checkups, you and your doctor will be more likely to catch such abnormalities.

The decision to discontinue HRT should be made in consultation with your doctor. It is not a good idea to simply stop, "cold turkey," unless it's a medical emergency; your body will probably go through an uncomfortable withdrawal phase. Some physicians recommend tapering off—perhaps taking the medication every other day at first, and gradually tapering down to nothing.

Dr. Karen Blanchard cautions that HRT is not something that should be started and stopped. A woman should not, in her opinion, say to herself, "'Gee, this month I'd like to not have hot flashes, so I'll take my estrogen,' and then say, 'I don't feel like taking it now, so I'll stop for a year or two. And if I start having problems with my bladder again, I'll take it for a few months or a couple of years and then I'll stop it again.' Taking estrogen on again/off again isn't wise and can, in fact, be more dangerous than beneficial in terms of osteoporosis.

"There is certainly danger to stopping and starting estrogen replacement therapy, because for the first three to five years after menopause, there's a very rapid drop-off in bone mass," Blanchard continues. "If you took estrogen and stopped it, took estrogen and stopped it, you could go through that phase many times, and, in fact, wind up with your bones in much worse shape than if you'd never taken it to begin with."

Explore Your Alternatives

No two women will respond alike to HRT. You need a physician who will treat your individual symptoms, not just prescribe standardized medications and dosages. Many women do fine on Premarin and Provera or another form of progesterone; others may fare better with the Estraderm patch and Provera. It's helpful to keep track of the symptoms you experience, so that you and your doctor can decide how to address them. And there are also steps you can take on your own.

Self-Help Tips

- For *fluid retention*—avoid excessive salt in your diet, avoid sugar when taking progestins, and increase vitamin B-6 from dietary or supplement sources.

- For *stomach upset*—take the medication at night with a light snack of bland food.

- For *depression* or *migraine headaches*—notify physician immediately.

- For *dizziness*—call your physician right away. Do not operate a car or machinery.

- For *trouble with your contact lenses*—report symptom to your prescribing physician and visit your ophthalmologist.

- For *discomfort with bleeding*—if everything checks out at your physical exam, ask your doctor whether you could take a combined estrogen-progestin dosage daily, and thus eliminate the monthly bleeding. The current PEPI Trial is evaluating how such a combined pill would affect the blood lipids (fats), but it won't be published until early 1995. However, two Danish researchers published a study in the December 1990 *British Journal of Obstetrics and Gynaecology* in which 49 women, separated into treatment and placebo groups, participated. They illustrated how such a combined therapy might work to both protect bone and keep cholesterol low. Although the drugs and dosages used were different from what is used here in the United States, they found that bone mineral content (BMC) was stable for the five years of treatment, whereas the placebo group lost 10% of BMC. In the hormone-taking group, total cholesterol and bad cholesterol decreased by 20%, whereas HDL was unchanged. So this therapy prevented bone loss completely, while also maintaining a lipid profile that is associated with prevention of coronary artery disease. That seems promising, although the sample of women studied was low and the medication dosages were different.

Combine Treatments?

Chapter Seven will explore some of the non-drug alternatives to HRT. However, it need not be a question of all or nothing with HRT. According to acupuncturist and Doctor of Oriental Medicine Diane Sandler, it's very common for naturopaths to treat women with herbal remedies while they are on estrogens. (You can read more about this in Chapter Seven.)

Or like Anita, whom you met in Chapter Four, you may have a physician who prescribes alternative medications. Anita began taking HRT after being amenorrheic for most of her adult life. Her physician was concerned about bone loss and about protecting Anita's endometrium with monthly periods. After several months on Premarin and Provera, Anita was having trouble adjusting to the hormones. She felt uncomfortable, experiencing breast swelling and tenderness and uterine tenderness. Her physician suggested switching her to Ogen, a synthetic form of estrogen. After 14 days on the new pill, Anita reports "so far, so good." The breast tenderness is gone, and she feels no adverse effects. In addition, Anita plans to try some acupuncture, with her physician's blessing, to help put her back in better balance.

Conclusion

Have you ever heard a friend tell you about being "put on" a medication? Women often talk about HRT using the same language: "My doctor put me on hormones." "My doctor put me on estrogen." What those phrases communicate, if we really listen to them, is the notion of the doctor knowing what's best for you, the patient. But for many of us, that notion is changing.

You can make the doctor-patient relationship a partnership situation by being attentive to your own body and symptoms. After all, it is you, with the help of your physician, who needs to make the estrogen decision. You know your own body best, and by listening to the signals your body sends, as well as getting all the information you can, you can make a difference in your own health care.

Remember, menopause is not a disease. It is a continuum of events that began way back before you were born, and if you use this time as an opportunity to find out more about your own health, it can be very productive.

A prescription for HRT is not set in stone. You do not automatically renew such a prescription—you must go in for a checkup first. This affords another opportunity for you, as a patient actively involved in your own health care, to discuss

the therapy with your doctor. HRT must be thoroughly discussed before it's begun *and* during regular visits to your
prescribing physician, whether he or she is your gynecologist,
internist, or family practitioner.

If it is your decision to proceed with hormone replacement, you may have quite a few questions about what that will
mean for you physically. You probably won't be able to feel
many of the physical benefits—such as the arresting of bone
loss or the raising of your good cholesterol level. Other effects
are, of course, quite noticeable—having a monthly period
again, for instance, or retaining water and gaining weight. Eva,
a 63-year-old retired teacher, doesn't notice anything different
at all while she's taking hormones. She has a monthly period
("Doesn't bother me a bit") and continues with her positive,
active life.

Some researchers estimate the number of postmenopausal
women on hormone replacement therapy at between 24% and
39%. But a 1990 study by Jane Cauley put the number of
women over 65 on estrogens at only 17%. Although the
number of estrogen prescriptions dispensed in the United
States rose from 14 million in 1980 to 20 million in 1986, it's
very hard to estimate the actual number of women who are
presently taking hormones. Many women stop taking them
when their major menopausal symptoms dissipate. Medical
experts speculate that the normal physical side effects of
HRT—most notably, bleeding, weight gain, and other minor
irritations—may be the reason that women do not stay on the
therapy.

So often we find that body and mind work together.
What's physical, what's psychological? In the next chapter
we'll explore the emotional aspects of menopause and hormone replacement therapy and learn how to deal with them.

6

Is it You or Your Hormones? The Emotional Consequences of Menopause and HRT

• • •

"My mother was 40 when I was born. I'm not sure exactly how old she was when she went through menopause, but I know I was about 10. It was wild. Our family is emotional anyway, but my mom became practically schizophrenic. Her emotions went up and down, and I was the butt of a lot of emotional and physical abuse. It didn't take much to set her off. I never talked to her about it, but in retrospect, I can see that the extremes of

her personality were exacerbated by the menopause.

"[When I think about menopause] I'm scared that I'll get out of control. I think I have more consciousness than my mother, and I have the feeling that my mother was much more indulgent in it. But when I was 27, I went off birth control pills—I had been on them for five years—and went through a seven-month depression. That experience, coupled with what I experienced with my mother, causes me to think I have a predisposition to be at the mercy of a genetic hormonal structure. I don't want to be that out of control. I also don't mind having my periods—I've never minded that much. I see it as sort of a womanly thing. So the dual threat of giving up menstruation and having this chamber of horrors that comes with it scares me."

—JENNIFER, age 40

We now know that besides hot flashes and cessation of menstrual periods, emotional symptoms can be one of the hallmarks of the menopause. As she moves into perimenopause and menopause, a woman may find herself much more susceptible to mood swings and more likely to cry for almost no reason, or to become more easily irritated. These are some of the menopausal symptoms that have led to harmful stereotyping of women. Women may become more emotionally unstable during this time, but getting to the scientific cause of it is not helped by characterizing menopausal women as harpies. The emotional side effects of menopause and the isolating nature of those stereotypes can contribute to a lot of discomfort for women and their families, as Jennifer remembers so well.

How can we differentiate between psychological problems and hormonal changes? When you're feeling upset, how do you determine what's really causing your emotional state? First of all, if you understand that there are physical reasons for your mood shifts and for feeling depressed or anxious during perimenopause and menopause, you can seek available treatments. Realizing that you are feeling this way *for a reason* may make the symptoms less threatening.

In this chapter, you'll meet women who have dealt with or are currently dealing with the emotional realities of the menopause and HRT. They will share some of the ways they have coped with their situations. Often the critical challenge in adjusting to the menopause, as with any other important passage in one's life, is simply to be heard and understood. This is also true if you've decided to start HRT, since the therapy can carry its own physical and emotional difficulties. But again, if you have a physician, family, and friends who will listen to you and can understand your concerns, that's the first step. There are ways to alleviate emotional difficulties and to make a smoother transition through menopause.

Melissa is a Santa Monica, California-based M.F.C.C. (Marriage, Family and Child Counselor) who specializes in women's empowerment issues and who works with survivors of physical and sexual abuse. She decided to start hormone replacement therapy because "I felt like I was bitchy, a little more forgetful, and just irritable and more glum," she recalls. "And a lot of that went away when I started on hormone replacement therapy." As a therapist and a menopausal woman, she is interested in exploring the issues connected with menopause as a turning point in a woman's life.

Whether or not you start hormone replacement therapy, awareness of the symptoms of menopause can help in your adjustment to it. In decades past, and certainly during the 1950s, when Jennifer's mother went through menopause, women often suffered needlessly because of the lack of knowledge about menopause. When women complained about their mood swings or irritability to their predominantly male doctors, they were often told, "It's all in your head." They were frequently prescribed tranquilizers, which can take care of the *symptoms* of depression but do nothing to address its causes. And indeed, since some tranquilizers act by reducing the overactivity of some nerve cells in the brain, they can actually decrease a woman's motivation to complain or seek out help. The wrong tranquilizer can even make someone more depressed.

According to Sonia Hamburger, clinical instructor at the University of California San Diego School for Reproductive Medicine's Menopause Education Clinic in La Jolla, California, the emotional side effects of menopause are often not well understood.

A crusader and advocate of women's health issues, Hamburger asserts that the medical establishment has finally begun to take menopause more seriously. "The interesting thing is that when osteoporosis became associated with menopause, we moved forward. Now we can have books with 'menopause' in the title! With the proliferation of articles and books on the menopause, I don't have to shout 'Menopause!' in crowded elevators any more," she laughs.

But old attitudes die hard. Despite a general acknowledgment on the part of the medical profession that menopause can cause emotional difficulties, women still have trouble getting their doctors to listen to them.

The Emotional Fallout from Hormonal Changes

Menopause causes profound changes in your body. As your levels of estrogens fall, your progesterone levels also shift. These hormonal fluctuations can cause a whole galaxy of physical symptoms, as well as symptoms that may *seem* to be emotional but that are really emotional manifestations of a chemical imbalance.

Although knowing there's a physical cause to which you can attribute emotional symptoms doesn't eradicate the emotional discomfort, it can be reassuring. For example, realizing her weepiness is caused by hormones allows a mother who's just given birth to understand why she's crying, and thus feel less "crazy." Being aware of the role hormones play in emotional outbursts can also help her spouse to be more understanding. Similarly, women who experience PMS often notify their spouses or boyfriends that if they appear more irritable than usual, it's because they're experiencing hormonal changes.

Conventional wisdom has it that women get depressed more often when they go through "the change." But scientific studies have not been able to establish that estrogen deficiency actually causes depression. However, Sonia Hamburger points out that "menopause for some women can be terribly stressful. And if the woman's response to stress in the past has been to become depressed, then she will often become depressed during menopause. But it's not directly caused by the menopause."

"I see a number of women who tell me, 'Gee, I'm having a tough time with menopause,' but they really are having a clinical depression," reports UCSD internist and reproductive endocrinologist Cynthia A. Stuenkel. Dr. Stuenkel gives a

Beck Inventory to her menopausal patients to fill out in the waiting room prior to their first full-hour consultation with her. This questionnaire is designed to help them (and her) separate out physical symptoms from the emotional ones. A woman can have feelings of loss about going through menopause and still not be clinically depressed, notes Stuenkel. Clinical depression is heralded by several distinct symptoms, and a list of them appears near the end of this chapter. This will give you some idea of whether counseling or therapy might be helpful in your situation.

This much is certain, though: When you go through natural or surgical menopause, your body responds to estrogen deprivation in a variety of ways. The most common symptom, experienced by 75% to 85% of all menopausal women, is the hot flash or flush. Besides a blood level establishing low estrogens and cessation of menstrual periods, this is the universal marker that a woman is entering menopause.

Even if hot flashes do not awaken a woman at night, her quality of sleep is still affected by insufficient estrogens—particularly the deep sleep (REM or rapid eye movement sleep time) that we require to feel sufficiently rested. And if you don't get good-quality sleep, you are less able to handle the stresses and problems of the next day. Sleep loss can make anyone feel cranky, depressed, and mentally confused.

Estrogen deprivation can also increase emotional variability, irritability, and loss of libido, or sex drive. Cathy, age 56, recalls that she started losing interest in sex right after her hot flashes began, right on target, at age 51. "I couldn't tell you whether it was just a physical reaction, of being uncomfortable and ill at ease with my body, or whether I was afraid of what all these changes meant—that I am getting older, flabbier, less attractive to my husband. But I just wasn't interested in having intercourse. It was really difficult for a couple of years. My husband didn't really understand what I was going through physically. My vagina got very dry and it was uncomfortable to have sex. I felt myself getting defensive, and he started getting more frustrated.

"Finally, we decided to try some couples therapy. We had been once before when the kids were in high school and we were having a lot of problems. Anyway, the therapists were husband and wife. We started talking about our sexual problems. They recommended a very good gynecologist, whom we both went to talk to. He did some additional blood work and found that my hormones were out of balance. He suggested estrogen therapy, which I agreed to try. And we continued to work on our problems in counseling. We're not there yet, but things are improving. And I think that being up-front about what I'm feeling is helping us communicate better."

The Cultural Pressures of Menopause

We heard about how Jennifer's mother's menopausal mood swings affected her own fears regarding menopause. But even when our mothers have an uneventful menopause, we often dread this passage because of the stigma society attaches to it. And to the degree that we internalize society's negative view of middle-aged women, we may anticipate emotional difficulties. Let's take a look at some of the cultural and personal pressures that intersect at this important time in a woman's life.

In earlier decades, menopausal women were labeled as unattractive and hysterical. Freda, 52, who was raised in Austria, recalls that in the "old days," before we understood what was happening biologically, women who couldn't cope with menopause were often labeled mentally ill and institutionalized!

As recently as 20 years ago, drug company estrogen ads in physicians' magazines tried to sell estrogen therapy by claiming it was an effective way to "manage" the cranky menopausal patient. A misunderstanding of what caused their symptoms made women feel even worse. They couldn't control what was happening to their bodies or their minds, yet they got criticism from their families, doctors, and society at large, making them feel even more isolated and helpless.

Today's menopausal woman is most likely working both outside and inside the home. She may still be raising children or, if she had children in her mid- to late 20s, going through the "empty nest syndrome." Her husband may be experiencing his own midlife crisis, and one or both of them are probably dealing with the care of aging parents. For these women, says Hamburger, "Menopause couldn't come at a worse time!" Added to lives that are already emotionally full to the brim, the stresses of hormonal changes can become the last straw. A strong support network is essential for coping with so many pressures.

Despite the women's movement and a more scientifically enlightened awareness concerning menopausal symptoms, this natural event in women's lives is still looked upon by our culture as disagreeable and depressing. Menopause signals that our "fruitful" life is over.

This continuum of events reminds us that we are not able to have children any longer. It is normal and acceptable to have feelings of loss and sadness about going through menopause. "I think psychologically it's a bummer," notes Nicky. "It signifies that you're changing and you're reaching another plateau in your life." Some of us may be reluctant about accepting the menopause because it reminds us that we are getting older. This society hasn't been kind to older women. Because of the emphasis placed on youth and beauty, we may fear that our husbands will leave us. And, in fact, this *does* happen to some middle-aged women. If a woman is single, she may worry that she will never be able to attract a man.

Mainstream physicians are beginning to look at the cultural component in a woman's adjustment to reproduction and menopause. In their textbook *Clinical Gynecologic Endocrinology and Infertility,* authors Leon Speroff, Robert H. Glass, and Nathan G. Kase ask the question, "Is PMS due to an individual pathologic problem or is it due to cultural beliefs, beliefs that lead to the menstrual cycle being associated with a variety of negative reactions? . . . What if our societies and cultures had celebrated menstruation as a time of pleasure (and even public joy) rather than something private (to be hidden) and negative? Would we have PMS today?" Would we have women reporting as many difficulties with menopause if this passage in a woman's life were likewise cause for celebration—as a time of maturation and wisdom? In fact, many women I talked with welcomed the end of their childbearing years and embraced middle age as a time when they were freer to choose how to live their lives.

But the feelings of loss are just as real and valid. And if a woman is able to first accept what this passage means in her life, and to mourn that loss, she may be able to make the transition better than by denying it. One of the best things you can do for yourself is to prepare for menopause by educating yourself about it. Dr. Stuenkel points out, "We show little girls movies when they're 10 and we say, 'You're a woman now, you're going to menstruate,' and then we leave it open-ended.

They anticipate they'll have babies, but no one tells them what happens at the other end of that reproductive spectrum.

"When I say to patients, 'Here's what I think is going on with you—you're going through the menopause,' they are able to handle it. But when they don't know why they are having symptoms and think that something else must be drastically the matter with them, it is frightening."

Menopause is different for every woman. It is estimated that only about 30% of women going through the menopause seek medical help for their symptoms. Because our physical health and emotional health are so inextricably linked, it is important for a woman to accept these changes and find help if she needs it. That may often be hard to do. "Women going through menopause are stressed for a number of reasons," notes Hamburger, "not the least of which is being put down by their doctors and having this constant sense that their bodies are telling them something but their doctors are pooh-poohing it."

Will the Doctor Listen?

You may have been one of millions of viewers who caught this 1991 episode of *thirtysomething,* an episode entitled "Life Class."*

Interior Doctor's Consultation Room—Day
Nancy waits. Doctor Eilertson enters, carrying a clipboard, upbeat, cheery . . .

EILERTSON
So! We're gonna talk about
changing your estrogen—?

114

Nancy looks right at him, and makes a decision.

                    NANCY
No.

                  EILERTSON
(barely grazed by this)
No? I thought—I just got off
the phone with Doctor
Silverman, she says we might
want to play with your
estrogen . . .

He waits. Nancy, weirdly, just stares at him.

                  EILERTSON
(beginning, just barely, to fray)
Okay?

                    NANCY
You want to *play* with my
estrogen?
Play with it? Why do you use
that word?

                  EILERTSON
(considerably cheered down)
It's just a word, Nancy.

---

*Script dialogue courtesy MGM Worldwide Television Group, a division of MGM-Pathé Communications Co.

When *thirtysomething* scriptwriter Winnie Holzman's show aired last year, she received a flood of letters from women viewers who told her, "I wish I could have said that to my doctor!" You too may have cheered for Nancy Weston as she spoke up to her doctor and told him that his words betrayed an attitude she would not accept as a patient. She refused to let him invalidate her.

As a woman, you may have identified with Nancy's frustration at trying to communicate with a physician who is not only disrespectful, but not attentive enough or too busy to fully listen to your concerns.

With the proliferation of HMOs (health maintenance organizations), where profit is made if health costs are kept down, women may find themselves shunted into busy clinic-like settings where the doctor cannot spend longer than 7 to 10 minutes at a stretch with any one patient. Even with private insurance coverage and the ability to choose your physician, you may still feel the squeeze for time. Because of high office rents, runaway malpractice insurance premiums and expensive equipment, physicians in private and group practices operate under enormous overheads. To make a profit, they need to see more patients every day.

These are the realities of our health-care system today. But there is another reality—your emotional state. And if you can't get a professional to listen to you, you may feel isolated and even a little "crazy": "Am I imagining this, or is this really happening to me? Why is it happening? Is it my hormones or my personality?"

As you approach menopause and begin to feel changes happening in your body, you are apt to run into a problem: finding a physician who will listen to your feelings about this life transition, and how you want to deal with it. Women may think that finding a female physician will take care of the problem, but it's not necessarily true. Nicky didn't find her female physicians any more caring than the male internist she had seen previously.

"What women don't need [during this time of transition] is to be put down," notes Sonia Hamburger, director of UCSD's Menopause Clinic. Whether your menopause is surgical or natural, you experience a tremendous physical and emotional upheaval.

Some women experience no emotional side effects when they go through menopause. Others aren't so lucky. Freda, 52, went through an early menopause 10 years ago and recalls, "I went through hell." Her mood swings were so severe, she says, that "at times I wouldn't have even cared if I'd gotten hit by a car. I was that miserable." What made Freda's situation even worse was that she had an old-fashioned doctor, a family physician who didn't believe in prescribing hormones. Freda is fine now, and says that she's back to feeling good again. "But nobody should have to go through what I went through," she says.

Marilyn, 47, has been on estrogens since the age of 31, when she had a complete hysterectomy. For many years, she complained to physicians that she had no libido and that she thought a hormone imbalance was responsible. No, they told her, that can't be. In fact, most women experience an increased sex drive after a hysterectomy, they said. Finally, she consulted a reproductive endocrinologist who tested her androgens (male hormones found in the ovaries that are precursors to the formation of estrogens) and found she had low levels of those hormones. Androgens are also responsible for sexual desire. To address this critical imbalance, Marilyn's doctor decided to supplement her estrogen prescription with testosterone. Marilyn is delighted that her desire for sex has come back, and relieved that she's finally found a physician with whom she can communicate.

A Plan of Action

If you're entering menopause, there are steps you can take to minimize emotional repercussions.

- *Talk with your doctor.* As in Marilyn's case, it is only after finding a doctor who will listen that you'll ultimately find an appropriate treatment. If your primary physician or gynecologist isn't well versed in reproductive endocrinology, you might want to ask him or her for a referral to a reproductive endocrinologist, a subspecialty in the field of gynecology which requires additional training and board certification.

- *Keep a diary.* Note the dates and length of your menstrual periods, how heavy or light the flow is, and other details. Also notate hot flashes—when they occur, for how long—and rapid or radical mood swings.

- *Get support.* Let your spouse and significant others know what you are going through. Obtain relevant literature and let them read it too. Explain to your children that you need some extra time for relaxing right now.

    Of course, if your symptoms are severe and you suspect that you may be clinically depressed, it's best to consult a professional counselor or psychotherapist. The Health Research Group of the Department of Health and Human Services cites several signposts that signal a need for mental health evaluation. Because emotional changes may indicate a physical disorder, and because menopause is inextricably linked with hormonal changes, you should have a complete physical examination to rule out a *physical* cause for your symptoms. Here are some of the signs of clinical depression:

- a change in sleeping or eating patterns *without obvious cause.*

- a sudden increase in or intolerable levels of anxiety, anger, or despair.

- feelings of extreme isolation, loneliness, or unhappiness.

- self-destructive urges or addictive behavior (such as abuse of alcohol or drugs).

- a change in sex drive. (It's *very* important to sort out physical versus emotional causes on this one during the menopause.)

- inability to function properly or to cope with ordinary routines.

- marked changes in mood from up to down, or prolonged periods of being too high or too low in mood.

- *Be a friend to yourself.* Many women tend to be very hard on themselves, expecting to be supermom, superwife, super career person. If you are comparing yourself to the Jane Fonda role model, "you're in real trouble," says Sonia Hamburger in UCSD Menopause Clinic sessions. Ease up on yourself. As my friend Melinda says, "I wouldn't talk to my *friends* the way I talk to myself sometimes!" Instead of focusing on what you *haven't* done, ask yourself what you need to feel better during this time. Maybe it's some time alone, time with a good friend, or time to get the exercise that might help you feel more relaxed. Then make a list and schedule those times into your week.

• *Be an advocate for your own health care.* During her educational lecture which introduces the afternoon-long session at UCSD's Menopause Clinic, Sonia Hamburger suggests that women draw on the skills they honed as mothers, when they were advocates for their children at the pediatrician's office. Schedule a consultation appointment with your physician *before* the onset of menopause to talk about what you should be prepared for—including emotional side effects.

Interview your doctor. Perhaps your ob/gyn is not really interested in or equipped to deal with menopausal women. Margie, whom you may remember from Chapter Three, found out that the clinic she had routinely visited for yearly Pap smears and birth control was only interested in treating women in their reproductive years. So she interviewed several practitioners until she found a group of female physicians who were set up to follow women through their later years as well.

- *Seek out a menopause clinic or menopause support group.* The camaraderie of being with other women experiencing the same transition in life can be extremely reassuring. At the University of San Diego Medical Center, bimonthly informal education sessions are held. For a nominal fee, women are given questionnaires about their range of symptoms, a two-hour talk about menopause, osteoporosis, and other related issues, and private counseling sessions in which they discuss their own symptoms. Later in the afternoon, a fellow in obstetrics and gynecology from the Medical Center visits and answers individual medical questions.

There are other such resources available throughout the country. The North American Menopause Society (NAMS), in addition to holding meetings for professionals, has materials and resources available to the public. Consult the list of resources listed at the back of this book. You can also call the Department of Reproductive Medicine at the nearest university or teaching hospital in your area. These departments often offer clinic visits for a nominal fee and you may be able to consult with the teaching physicians on staff.

Research about women's health, and reproductive health in particular, is currently going through an expansion period. The National Institutes of Health, now headed by Bernadine Healy, M.D., has established a Women's Health Initiative which will encompass innumerable research projects on all aspects of women's health into the next century. This is a good time for women. We know more than previous generations did about how our bodies work, and we have the consciousness to ask questions and seek the proper support. Menopause is no longer an event to be hidden away. We can bring it out of the closet and help ourselves deal with all the changes, positive and negative.

Hormone replacement therapy affords tremendous relief to women going through the menopause. However, your symptoms may not be that debilitating. Accordingly, you may decide that HRT is not for you, or that its risks outweigh its benefits. The next chapter offers a variety of alternative therapies and self-help tips, as substitutes or supplements to HRT.

7

Alternatives
to HRT

• • •

*"The reason American women don't know hot
flashes are easy to deal with is because they don't
really know much about Chinese medicine. . . .
When the kidney energy is strong, you don't have
hot flashes, and you have strong bones."*
—SUSAN LANGE,
Doctor of Oriental Medicine, Meridian Center,
Santa Monica, California

Perhaps you have doubts about taking hormones during menopause or, for that matter, for the rest of your life. You may have a family history of breast cancer or be concerned by the inconclusiveness of studies about estrogens and the link with breast cancer. Or maybe you're just not a pill-taker. If you have such reservations, you're not alone. There are naturopathic practitioners and women's health advocacy groups who maintain that when it comes to the menopause, most women can manage their symptoms naturally, using diet, supplements, and exercise.

Joanne, now 53, recalls going through "three years of hell and the whole transition of aging" during her menopause. "I was so sad about the loss of my period," she says. "It had been a hassle, but somehow it was always a welcome part of my biology. When I started going through menopause, I wondered if my femininity really depended on my fertility."

She was suffering from other symptoms too. Although she'd always been thin, she was putting on weight, and she was having hot flashes that were "unbearable and getting worse." Joanne began taking estrogens to cope with the hot flashes. But then something else started to happen. "After a year and a half I felt as though my fingernails weren't growing any more. The same thing had happened when I was on birth control pills for six years. Of course, there's no way to document whether the estrogen was causing that or whether it was my imagination. But I decided to go off estrogen and about a month later the hot flashes came back."

That's when she met Susan Lange, a Doctor of Oriental Medicine at the Meridian Center in Santa Monica, California. Joanne began working with Dr. Lange, who is an acupuncturist and expert in Chinese herbs. "Basically, the treatment was to strengthen the liver and the kidneys. Everything Susan did for the first six months was supportive and cleansing."

Dr. Lange also encouraged Joanne, who had been teaching aerobics prior to her treatment, to stop doing any vigorous physical exercise. "My energy had run out and I was developing this pain in my left hip," recalls Joanne. "It was all I could do just to walk my dogs. Susan just kept saying, 'Listen to your body, listen to your body.' So I *stopped* all exercise. It was very, very difficult because I had always thought exercise was good for you. [With the use of herbs and acupuncture], it took me six months to get my stamina up. Then, suddenly, I started being able to do things, and now I have all this energy again."

For some women, taking charge of their health means eschewing mainstream doctors and seeking out alternative healing practices. Although Chinese medicine has been practiced for thousands of years in the East, the Western world has been slow to embrace these healing philosophies and techniques. If you decide to work with this method of healing, you will find a very different base of assumptions at work. According to practitioners such as Luc De Schepper, a Los Angeles–based M.D. and licensed acupuncturist, Western medicine often relies solely on pharmacology and invasive techniques to heal the body. In the Chinese model of medicine, on the other hand, each emotion is linked to an organ; if there is an imbalance in that organ, deficiency and illness can result. Eastern medicine assumes that by restoring the body's balance, the energy in the body is released to do its own healing. In this chapter, we'll look at what natural methods can and cannot do for you. And in the final section, I'll talk about current studies using alternative drugs to deal with the threat of osteoporosis.

Menopause: Disease or Passage?

Women's health-care advocates object strenuously to the characterization of menopause as a disease (estrogen deficiency) that must be managed medically (hormone replacement therapy). Author Susanne Morgan, in her book *Coping with a Hysterectomy,* charges that drug companies "have 'created' menopause as an 'estrogen deficiency disease'" and used it as a marketing strategy to sell more medication. She and other advocates contend that for most women menopause causes minimal discomfort, and that a woman's body, if allowed, can make enough endogenous estrogen to carry her through and beyond the menopause. They argue that women can utilize non-drug alternatives to deal with their symptoms and that therefore hormones are unnecessary.

Menopause is not a disease, of course, but profound endocrine and bodily changes occur during the climacteric (the period from perimenopause to cessation of menopausal symptoms). Interestingly, the word *climacteric* comes from *klimakter*, a Greek word meaning "rung of the ladder," a critical point in human life. The climacteric signals a particular passage in a woman's life: the gradual cessation of reproduction. As such, it presents a variety of symptoms and changes. There are ways to deal with it in a commonsense manner, and to take advantage of the opportunities it presents. Listed below are the most common effects of the menopause and suggestions for dealing with them. You can make use of these techniques with or without HRT.

Common Complaints, Commonsense Approach

The most pronounced, direct, and immediate symptoms of menopause are hot flashes, vaginal dryness, urinary discomforts, and stress. Let's take a look at commonsense approaches to each one.

Hot Flashes

Hot flashes are not a hazard to your health, but they can be debilitating if severe enough. According to current theory, the hot flash is not a release of body heat, but a "sudden, inappropriate excitation of heat release mechanisms" [Speroff et al., *Clinical Gynecological Endocrinology and Infertility*]. The hot flash coincides with a surge of LH (luteinizing hormone). Women usually feel an aura of warmth just before it happens, and although the surface of the body heats up, the body's interior, or core temperature, falls.

Although scientists still do not completely understand what triggers them, hot flashes are not imagined, they are real. Ask any woman who has experienced them.

For some women, it is simply a matter of opening a window or going outside for a brief time until the symptom passes. (Episodes can last anywhere from a few seconds to several minutes.) If hot flashes bother you during the daytime, it's a good idea to dress in layers. That way, if you feel a flush coming on, you can simply take off a sweater or outer garment. However, severe hot flashes produce profuse sweating and require a change of clothing. Although there are no scientific data to support it, taking vitamin E (30 to 60 IU, or international units) has been helpful to many women in reducing the intensity of hot flashes. There are also some herbal remedies, teas, and other preparations that anecdotal evidence suggests can offer relief. (See the herbal remedies section later in this chapter.)

Vaginal Dryness

Along with flattening of the breasts, hot flashes, and lessening of menstrual periods comes vaginal dryness. As your vaginal walls become thinner and less moist, intercourse can become quite painful—a condition known as dyspareunia. And that can have serious consequences for your sex life.

127

Nicky's gynecologist recommended a fantastic lubricant, called Astro Glide™, which helps with the dryness that comes with menopause. For years, K-Y Jelly™ has been a standard lubricant, but some object to its gumminess. You may want to experiment with different lubricants (such as Replens™) on the market. Just make sure you don't use petroleum jelly—it coats your tissues so they can't breathe, and becomes a breeding ground for bacteria.

Estrogen creams also relieve vaginal dryness, but don't make the mistake of assuming that inserting an estrogen suppository is different from taking hormones. There are many blood vessels in your vagina and the hormones will be readily absorbed into your bloodstream. You also need to be aware that using estrogen cream too close to intercourse can also affect your partner, causing potential irritation of the penis and delivering the hormone to his system as well. One study, for instance, documented growth of breast tissue in male subjects who had received estrogens as part of their cancer treatment.

Some sources recommend regular sexual activity as the panacea to vaginal dryness ("use it or lose it"). But of course it's the question of which comes first, the cart or the horse. If your vagina is dry and you experience pain with penetration, then you're less likely to desire more sex with your partner.

Urinary Symptoms

Once you go through menopause, estrogen receptors in your bladder and urinary tract are no longer replenished, causing an increased likelihood of urinary incontinence and susceptibility to urinary infection.

Health-care practitioners recommend doing Kegel exercises to strengthen the base of the bladder and urethra. These exercises are beneficial for women of all ages and especially for postpartum and menopausal women. Simply squeeze with your vaginal muscles as if you're trying to hold back urinating. Repeat this squeezing 10 to 20 times, up to 5 times a day. Many women report a lessening of stress incontinence when they do these exercises often. (Stress incontinence means losing urine when you cough, sneeze, or laugh. It is very common after vaginal delivery, because of the extra stress put on the bladder floor from pushing. It is also a consequence of aging.)

Dealing with Stress

"I see so many patients now who have early meno-pause. They come in and tell me, 'Listen, my mother did not have one hot flash until she was 52. I'm 41—what's going on?' I tell them, 'Your mother didn't live under the stress that you do. Chances are she wasn't trying to be both a mother and a career woman.'"
—JANET ZAND, O.M.D., Lic. Ac.,
Pacific Palisades, California

Is it true that women in general are going through menopause at an earlier age? Not according to mainstream physicians, who point out that the average age of menopause is still 51. But alternative physicians—including naturopaths and acu-puncturists, are perhaps seeing more women who have not gotten satisfaction from mainstream physicians and want to know what's causing their bodies to be out of balance. Whenever a woman goes through the climacteric, she can certainly experience added stresses, especially if the changes in her

129

hormonal system produce symptoms that interfere with her daily life.

For the last two decades the popular press has dealt extensively with the toll on health exacted by our modern lives. And yet just knowing that too much pressure from job, home, and family is deleterious to your health may not be enough to motivate you to change. Sometimes it takes an added stress to push us over the edge and make us realize it's time to make some changes.

The menopause can be the perfect opportunity to sit down and consider, either alone or with your partner and family, how to get through this time. Especially if you are feeling anxious and depressed, now is the time to do something about it.

The commonsense approach to stress is to lighten your load. Delegate some responsibilities. Are you overseeing too many household chores that could be handled by other family members? Are you overly concerned with having a perfectly neat house, when it might be better for your health to let go of certain details? Would it be worth it to hire someone to help out with some of the housework?

It may be helpful to look at the other arenas of your life and reevaluate pressures there too. For instance, are you driving yourself too hard at the office? Have you taken on too many outside responsibilities—with your church, PTA, civic and professional groups? It's a good idea to cut down on obligations and activities and devote more time to relaxation, exercise, and just plain fun!

Even though psychological symptoms are not actually caused by menopause, they may result from the extra stress you're subjected to during this time in your life. When you're feeling pressured and overloaded, that's a good sign that you need to acknowledge and pay attention to those stressors. Later

130

in the chapter we'll discuss relaxation techniques that can help to alleviate daily stress.

Of course, if your symptoms are severe and you suspect that you may be clinically depressed, it's best to consult a professional counselor or psychotherapist. Chapter Six listed several symptoms that may indicate you could be suffering from depression.

Beyond Menopause: Start Preparing Now

As you know, it's not just the acute symptoms of menopause that have doctors and health-care practitioners concerned. It's the long-range projections about heart and bone disease that are most worrisome. But should these two life-threatening diseases concern the majority of women? Sidney M. Wolfe, M.D., director of the Public Citizen Health Research Group in Washington, D.C., maintains that mortality-rate projections by epidemiologists are just a smokescreen for marketing estrogens to women who are otherwise perfectly healthy. You and your doctor will be the ones to decide whether this applies to you, and the next chapter will help you assess your own benefit-risk ratio.

But if you think your decision will be *against* hormone replacement therapy, it's a good idea to assess your health picture before the onset of menopause. As Dr. Janet Zand points out, "The best way to diminish your [menopausal] symptoms and to deal with osteoporosis is to take preventative measures. I really think women should begin at the age of 30. It makes good sense to have already instituted those habits before coming into perimenopause, because it takes time for nature to make a difference." What are some of the measures you could start today that will help your future health?

Your Bones: Don't Rob the Bank

One of your first lines of defense against bone loss is to have stronger bones before age 35, when all people, men and women, start to lose bone mass. Although the FDA (U.S. Food and Drug Administration) has established a minimum daily requirement of 800 mg of calcium for nonpregnant women, the National Osteoporosis Foundation recommends 1,000 mg daily for premenopausal women and 1,500 mg daily for menopausal and postmenopausal women. But results from the National Health and Nutrition Examination Survey II and others have shown that most middle-aged women only get between 400 and 500 mg a day of calcium.

How can you make sure you get 1,000 mg a day of calcium? Most experts agree that dietary sources are preferable to supplements. Three glasses of milk would do the trick. But for various reasons, that may not be the route you'll want to choose. Some people are lactose intolerant, which means that the sugars in milk do not agree with their digestive systems. Lactaid™ and Dairy Ease™, products found in supermarkets and pharmacies, replace the enzyme lactase that your body needs to digest milk. They're available as chewable tablets or as substitute milk products to be added to the milk you drink.

But you may also be staying away from dairy products for health reasons. Those trying to limit their cholesterol intake, to prevent heart disease and breast cancer (which studies now link to high-fat diets), are cautioned to reduce or eliminate the animal fats found in dairy products. You could

What Are Good Sources of Calcium?

Food	Selected Serving Size	Percentage of U.S. RDA[1]

BREADS, CEREALS, AND OTHER GRAIN PRODUCTS

English muffin, plain with
raisins .... 1 .... +
Muffin, bran .... 1 medium .... +
Oatmeal, instant, fortified,
prepared[2] .... ⅔ cup .... +
Pancakes, plain, fruit,
buckwheat, or whole-wheat 2 4-inch pancakes ... +
Waffles:
  Bran, cornmeal, or fruit . . 2 4-inch squares .... +
  Plain .... 2 4-inch squares .... + +

VEGETABLES

Broccoli, cooked .... ½ cup .... +
Spinach, cooked .... ½ cup .... +
Turnip greens, cooked .... ½ cup .... +

MEAT, POULTRY, FISH, AND ALTERNATES

Fish and Seafood
  Mackerel, canned, drained . 3 ounces .... +
  Ocean perch, baked or
    broiled .... 3 ounces .... +
  Salmon, canned, drained .. 3 ounces .... +

Dry Beans, Peas, and Lentils
  Tofu (bean curd)[3] .... ½ cup cubed .... + +

MILK, CHEESE, AND YOGURT

Cheese, natural:
  Blue, brick, camembert,
    feta, gouda, monterey,
    mozzarella, muenster,
    provolone, or roquefort . 1 ounce .... +

Food	Selected Serving Size	Percentage of U.S. RDA[1]
Cheese, natural (continued):		
Gruyere or swiss	1 ounce	+ +
Parmesan (hard) or romano	1 ounce	+ +
Cheese, process, cheddar or swiss	¾ ounce	+
Cheese, ricotta	½ cup	+ +
Ice cream or ice milk, soft-serve	½ cup	+
Milk:		
Buttermilk	1 cup	+ +
Chocolate	1 cup	+ +
Dry, nonfat, reconstituted	1 cup	+ +
Evaporated, whole or skim, diluted	1 cup	+ +
Lowfat or skim	1 cup	+ +
Whole	1 cup	+ +
Yogurt:		
Flavored or fruit, made with whole or lowfat milk	8 ounces	+ +
Frozen	8 ounces	+ +
Plain:		
Made with whole milk	8 ounces	+ +
Made with lowfat or nonfat milk	8 ounces	+ + +

[1]A selected serving size contains—
+   10-24 percent of the U.S. RDA for adults and children over 4 years of age
+ +   25-39 percent of the U.S. RDA for adults and children over 4 years of age
+ + + 40 percent or more of the U.S. RDA for adults and children over 4 years of age

See section on fortified foods.

If made with calcium sulfate.

Note: U.S. RDA (Recommended Daily Allowance) is not necessarily equal to the Minimum Daily Requirement. RDA may be higher (up to 1,200 mg daily) for postmenopausal women, according to other sources.

Reprinted with permission from U.S. Department of Agriculture, copyright Jan. 1990.

drink nonfat milk, which has just as much calcium. Or refer to the chart "What Are Good Sources of Calcium?", where you'll find nondairy dietary sources of calcium. The problem is, you have to eat an awful lot of broccoli to equal the calcium in just one glass of skim milk!

That leaves supplements. Dr. Robert Lindsay, director of the Regional Bone Center at the Helen Hayes Hospital in upstate New York, has done extensive research into osteoporosis and recommends taking a 200 mg supplement three times a day, with each meal. The calcium, which should be in the form of calcium carbonate, is better absorbed in lower doses and will remain at a steady level in your blood that way. Don't forget that you also need normal levels of vitamin D to absorb calcium. You can usually get enough just from being outside for a few minutes each day, since your body manufactures vitamin D when exposed to sunlight. Many food products also have added vitamin D, or you can safely take a 400-unit supplement each day in a multivitamin.

Another way to keep your body's calcium savings account solvent is to avoid the account drainers—alcohol, caffeine, and nicotine. All interfere with the absorption of calcium, which means calcium will be withdrawn from your bones to keep the blood level high enough.

Establishing a consistent exercise routine also assures continued bone strength. This means 20 to 30 minutes of sustained weight-bearing exercise three times a week: walking, jogging, weight training, dance classes, or high- or low-impact aerobics. If you're a swimmer, you're getting a good cardiovascular workout—but since your body is weightless you won't be building bone. Try to alternate your swimming routine with another weight-bearing activity, or take a water calisthenics ("Aquasize") class, which pits your muscles against the resistance of the water.

Bone loss can set you up for osteoporosis, when bones become lacy and brittle. But as health-care advocates point out, it's *falling* that actually causes the debilitating fractures of hip, wrist, and forearm that plague older women. Instead of relying on hormones to stabilize bone, they advocate prevention techniques aimed at reducing falls in the elderly. These techniques make good common sense for anyone:

- Avoid excessive alcohol. Even moderate amounts (2 glasses of wine per day) are not metabolized as quickly as you age.

- Avoid unnecessary medications, since incorrect or combined medications can produce dizziness and mental confusion.

- Have your vision checked regularly. Blurry vision or incorrect depth perception can result in a fall.

- Make sure floors are not slippery and that rugs are securely fastened down.

Guarding Your Heart

Women and heart disease: the AHA (American Heart Association) calls it the silent epidemic. Large studies of women—the Nurses' Health Study (32,000 postmenopausal women) and the Leisure World Study (8,881 postmenopausal women) showed that women taking estrogens had a 70% and 50% reduction, respectively, in heart attack risk over the women who didn't take them. If you don't want to take estrogens, does this mean you're doomed to get heart disease? No, and here's why: Keeping your overall cholesterol level below 200 mg/dl (milligrams per deciliter of blood), your HDL level over 35 mg/dl, and your LDL level below 130 mg/dl will reduce your risk of heart attack considerably.

Moderate, consistent aerobic exercise will also help to keep your cholesterol levels within range. Not smoking and low alcohol intake are, of course, primary prevention techniques. And should these lifestyle habits fail to bring your cholesterol levels within range, there are a variety of other medications that lower blood cholesterol levels very effectively. Presumably, though, if you've got objections to hormone replacement therapy, you don't really want to be on daily medications of any kind. A growing number of naturopathic practitioners have their own opinions—and solutions—to this very issue.

Herbal and Naturopathic Remedies

John P. Rodino, Ph.D., director of Bionutritional Consultants in Westminster, California, has a couple of objections to HRT: its carcinogenic potential and the standard dosages. He refers to a recent news story about a group of Orange County oncologists who are promoting tamoxifen, a chemotherapeutic agent that destroys estrogens. Those oncologists state that "by destroying estrogen in the female, you reduce her risk of cancer. Now, if destroying a female's estrogen reduces the risk of cancer, what would be the result of *increasing* a female's estrogen?"

Rodino also believes that the dosages of estrogens given are way too high. The average Premarin dose is .625 mg a day, which is equal to about 18 birth control pills a day. [A typical dosage of estrogen in Ortho-Novum contraceptive pills is .035.] And he thinks the rationale behind HRT is faulty: "I view estrogen as a reproductive hormone. There's a feeling in medicine that to be female requires estrogen. This concept of females needing estrogens forever is beyond me. Especially when you have this tremendous amount of evidence about how destructive estrogens can be carcinogenically."

Janet Zand, naturopathic physician, points out that some women can take HRT and do fine, "but those are the women I hardly ever see in my practice. The women who come to my office are women who have a history of breast cancer in their family or ovarian cancer or uncertain Pap results, and are scared to take a hormone." Zand also believes that the way estrogen is delivered in this country is inappropriate. "I think ultimately we're going to find out that less is more—that instead of a standard .625 mg dose, a woman might be able to take that every other day, or that the dose might be cut in half. As we become more sensitive to the actual needs of the female, we're going to reconstruct the format that we currently use. Right now it's functional, but I don't think it's harmonious with the female body. I treat many women who are on HRT, and the hormones have gotten rid of their hot flashes. But the other symptoms may linger, and herbal medicine, acupuncture, and homeopathy can often eliminate those."

Doctor of Oriental Medicine Susan Lange maintains that women don't need to take estrogens, either for short-term relief of hot flashes or for long-term prevention of osteoporosis. "The reason American women don't know hot flashes are easy to deal with is because they don't really know much about Chinese medicine. In Chinese medicine, the kidneys aren't just the organs we think of in Western medicine. They are connected with the essence you're born with, they're connected with your reproductive cycle, starting with menstruation all the way through menopause. They are also connected with memory, rejuvenation, and bones. When the kidney energy is strong, you don't have hot flashes, and you have strong bones." Lange works with her female patients to clear the kidneys through the use of Chinese herbs and acupuncture. And in so doing, she is able to restore their health and energy and diminish hot flashes.

Like many other Doctors of Oriental Medicine, Zand is partial to the plant world. The hundreds of peri- and postmenopausal patients she treats have responded well to *dong quai,* an "adaptogenic" herb that contains **phyto-estrogens** (plant estrogens), used in the Orient to treat the hot flashes, anxiety, depression, and insomnia that accompany menopause. According to Zand, adaptogenic herbs stimulate the body's immune system to encourage self-regulation. For example, an adaptogenic herb like ginseng will help lower the blood sugar in a hyperglycemic person. The same herb given to a person with hypoglycemia (very low blood sugar) will help bring the blood sugar level up.

Most women require additional herbs, such as *Agnus castus,* wild yam, and Siberian ginseng, in combination with the *dong quai* to ease their symptoms. Other herbs are often given to help detoxify the liver, since a sluggish liver is also a common cause of menopausal symptoms. Red raspberry leaf tones the uterus, but is not essential for all menopausal women.

In addition, says Zand, "I feel that there are certain dietary rules a menopausal woman would do well to follow. Choosing fruit instead of sugar; baked or steamed foods instead of fried foods; avoiding alcohol; and going easy on the salt are things that one would normally do to create a healthy diet. But they're even more important during menopause, because we're so vulnerable to stress during this time, and eating healthy helps us cope more easily with stress.

"Some rules are so basic, they're almost idiotic sounding, like 'don't eat unless you're hungry.' A lot of menopausal women tend to get more nervous and eat when they're not hungry, which produces another whole set of problems." According to Zand, avoiding sugar, red meat, chocolate, caffeine, and carbonated sodas will also help. The heavy concentrations of fats in red meat, for instance, can clog the digestive system, as will eating too much sugar.

"Menopause is so chaotic. You get your period in March and then you don't get it again until June. And your hormones do an Irish jig in between. That can be very trying. Anything that you can do to ritualize and organize your routines is helpful. Your routine will help to sustain you and get you through the tough, irregular times of menopause."

Plants are preferred by naturopaths because they are milder than drugs. For instance, *dong quai* contains plant estrogens that are 1/400th as strong as pharmaceutical dosages. Acupressurist Catherine Bauer, based in Oakland, California, also recommends *dong quai,* drunk as a tea before bedtime. She also praises motherwort to help regulate body temperature: One teaspoon of the leaves is steeped in one-half cup boiling water for 10 minutes. (A half-cup a day is the maximum, advises Bauer.) For urinary incontinence, Bauer recommends marshmallow root: Steep one cup of dried root in one cup boiling hot water and drink 1 to 2 cups a day.

A word of caution: Just because something is an herb and considered "natural" doesn't mean it cannot have a pharmacological effect. Whatever you take orally passes through your liver and is metabolized there. We don't know exactly what long-term effects these herbal remedies have. Unfortunately, most of the evidence about plant estrogens and herbal remedies is anecdotal.

Zand regrets the lack of scientific evidence. "There's very little money in this country for such research. The only way that I know if a woman is doing well is anecdotally. I treat her and then send her off to get a bone density study. And if her bones are still looking good, then I say, 'So far, so good.'" It's a good idea, if you want to embark on alternative remedies, to be working with a practitioner who's skilled in this arena.

Acupuncture, Acupressure

The Far East has given us other healing techniques as well. Both acupuncture and acupressure have gained acceptance in the United States in the last 10 years. Based on the Taoist philosophy that your life energy flows through your body in 12 defined paths, or meridians, the practice is based on ancient Chinese methods for freeing the energy when it becomes blocked along those pathways. Anita mentioned to her doctor that she wanted to try acupuncture to see if that would help her feel more balanced and alleviate some of the HRT symptoms she was experiencing. Her doctor agreed that it would be a good avenue to try.

You may already have tried these methods and found them helpful. They may be of even greater value during the climacteric, and many women report a good response from the treatments.

Other stress-reduction techniques, such as biofeedback and hypnosis, have found their way into mainstream medicine. Each of these methods can teach you to relax and to give yourself positive, helpful messages.

Non-Estrogen Drugs that May
Prevent Osteoporosis

There are several current studies investigating alternative ways to build bone. In women unable or unwilling to take estrogens, *calcitonin* is one possibility. It appears to inhibit further bone loss in cases of established osteoporosis, and is being tried in the forms of injection or nasal spray. However, right now it is being used on an investigational basis only; the FDA has not yet approved it for general use. If you are interested in exploring this possibility, contact the nearest university medical center to see if their gerontology department has any ongoing studies.

Etidronate, one of the bisphosphonate compounds, appears to decrease bone resorption, stabilize bone mass, and decrease spinal compression fractures. So far, those given the compound in studies over a period of two years have experienced minimal side effects. Etidronate has been approved by the FDA for treating Paget's bone disease, but not yet for treating osteoporosis in the general population.

In addition, there are ongoing trials attempting to find pharmaceutical agents not just to stop bone loss, but to stimulate the formation of new bone. *Fluoride* does stimulate the formation of one form of bone cell called an osteoclast, but its side effects of gastrointestinal upset and joint pains (arthralgias) have remained a problem. Dr. Robert Lindsay is studying parathyroid hormone to determine whether it can increase bone mass, but results won't be available until 1993.

Tamoxifen, an oral antiestrogen used in the treatment of breast cancer, may also be useful in preventing bone loss. Preliminary study results point to increased bone density as one of the positive side effects of this drug, which is now involved in a large government-sponsored drug trial to assess whether it can prevent breast cancer.

As you've seen in this chapter, there are a variety of alternative ways to deal with the menopause and with preventing osteoporosis and heart disease. The choices are yours. Some measures—from following a healthy diet and exercise plan to reducing the pressures and obligations in your life—make good common sense and don't cost a lot of money. You may want to explore further and seek out naturopathic practitioners with knowledge of Oriental medicine and healing methods, or keep abreast of research on non-estrogen drugs that may prevent osteoporosis.

Just as you must carefully choose your physicians and your own treatment methods, so must you carefully choose alternative methods. Whatever your decision about HRT, you must take an active role in building your own health.

For Further Reading:

Catherine Bauer, *Acupressure for Women*. The Crossing Press, Freedom, CA, 1987.

Sadja Greenwood, M.D., *Menopause Naturally*. Volcano Press, Volcano, CA, 1989.

Susanne Morgan, *Coping With a Hysterectomy—Your Own Choice, Your Own Solutions*. The Dial Press, New York, 1982.

Rosetta Reitz, *Menopause: A Positive Approach*. Penguin Books, New York, 1981.

Judith Sachs, *What Every Woman Should Know About Menopause.* Dell Medical Library, New York, 1991.

Gail Sheehy, *The Silent Passage: Menopause.* Random House, New York, 1992.

Wolf Utian, M.D., and Ruth S. Jacobowitz, *Managing Your Menopause.* Prentice Hall, New York, 1990.

8

Determining Your Own Benefit-Risk Ratio

. . .

"At first, when I started having hot flashes, I could predict that I would have one just after dinner. Then they went away for a while. Then I started having periods again. But now I'm <u>definitely</u> menopausal. I'm having hot flashes more often and more unpredictably. I decided I was going to try to do without hormones unless something drastic happens. I don't want my periods to go on and on, and I've always tended to do things more naturally. Our family practitioner is a former ob/gyn, and he's recommending that I <u>not</u> take hormones. He checked my bones, which he said were real good. That's not a surprise to me—I've always drunk milk. I know I'm starting to go through the menopause, but it's very mild so far. I have hot flashes and it's a little disconcerting, but

*it doesn't really bother me. I just take off my
sweater or open a window, and in five to ten minutes it passes. Hormones? I've decided to wait."*
— NANCY, age 49½

*"It's interesting. I started making inquiries [about
hormone replacement] after the fact. I went
through menopause, I seemed fine, and at all my
other checkups nobody said anything. When I complained to my internist about pain in my leg, he
said it was from being overweight. But when I
went to my daughter-in-law's gynecologist, she
sent me for a bone density X-ray and discovered
that I have osteoporosis in my leg. So she put me
on hormones. I was a little nervous about it, but I
had been suffering with my leg pain. I figured
since I have pain and this is going to occur with
other bones, wonderful, I'll do something about it.
So I was really glad to start. I think I feel a lot better now—I don't know whether it's because mentally I feel better, or whether it's due to the
hormones I'm taking."*
— PHYLLIS, age 62

Sooner or later, most American women, whether perimenopausal, menopausal, or postmenopausal, will probably hear their physicians suggest hormone replacement
therapy. The suggestion may have already caught you off
guard.

What are your choices? Your risks? Your benefits? You
need to carefully consider your own benefit-risk ratio and
discuss it, as well as your fears, with your own doctor. The

good thing about this medical decision is that it needn't be made in a hurry. Unless you're facing an imminent hysterectomy, you have time, especially if you begin now.

Each woman brings her own personal health and family health histories to her estrogen decision. Remember Debbie from Chapter Four? She's 44 and already going through an early menopause. She would like the benefits and advantages that HRT has to offer in helping her cope with menopausal symptoms. Her physician has told her that she should start thinking about HRT. But with a paternal grandmother who had breast cancer, she's just not sure what she should do. Maureen, who's in her late 40s, is planning to start hormone replacement when she becomes menopausal. Her risk factors for HRT are low, and she has had two friends who benefitted from the therapy by experiencing diminished hot flashes.

You may have strong concerns and definite opinions about HRT already, as does Nancy. But it may help your own deliberations to understand some of the thinking behind the present push for HRT. Why is HRT being recommended so highly? It's because evidence has been mounting in the last two decades for its protective effects in preventing osteoporosis and heart disease. In addition, estrogens offer the immediate and obvious benefits of alleviating the hot flashes and vaginal atrophy and dryness that come with menopause.

As an example of what materials your physician may have in mind when recommending HRT, consider the following excerpt from a June 1986 technical bulletin published by the American College of Obstetricians and Gynecologists:

The symptoms and risk factors of each patient must be evaluated individually, but every woman who has developed ovarian failure should be considered for estrogen

147

*replacement therapy [underlining added for emphasis].
Replacement therapy should be directed toward the relief of hot flushes [also called flashes] and atrophic
vaginitis, as well as the prevention of osteoporosis.
Protection against heart disease is also a benefit. Prevention of osteoporosis and heart disease require
long-term estrogen therapy.*

The ACOG's Technical Bulletin summarizes the pro-
HRT beliefs of the mainstream medical profession. Even for
those women who flat out do not want to take hormones, their
physicians will probably still try to offer education about the
short- and long-term benefits of HRT. Dr. Carolyn Kaplan, a
reproductive endocrinologist in Santa Monica, California,
states, "I have patients who are in menopause but who come
in telling me, 'There's no way you're going to get me to take
that estrogen.' Certainly in that situation I'm not about to try
to twist somebody's arm, but what I try to do is educate people
and let them assess their own benefit-risk ratio. I think it's
really a matter of quality of life."

No one is going to force you to take hormones. In fact,
surveys have shown that almost 50% of women who begin
HRT during the menopause stop taking them. But there are a
number of good reasons why you might want to consider
taking them, perhaps for as long as 20 years. The decision rests
with you and your physician, and this chapter is designed to
help you sort through your own individual benefit-risk ratio.

The decision about HRT really boils down to weighing
the Big Three reasons *for* the therapy—Menopausal Symptoms (for short-term, immediate benefits), Osteoporosis, and
Heart Disease (for long-term, quality-of-life benefits)—against
the One Serious reason *not* to take it: Breast Cancer (the most

feared yet still not clearly established risk). Of course, there are some women for whom HRT is absolutely contraindicated, and you'll find that list later in the chapter.

How do you balance your own benefit-risk factors in all of this? Sometimes it may feel as if you can't win for losing. A case in point: You're aware that to reduce your risk of heart disease, you need to keep weight off and cut down on your consumption of animal fats. But to keep your bones strong, you need to consume at least 1,000 mg of calcium daily, preferably from dietary sources. Dairy products, notorious for their fat content, are the first-line choices, but then you'd be adding pounds in order to keep your bones strong. On the other hand, according to experts, if you have a few extra pounds on your frame, it can't hurt in terms of protecting against osteoporosis!

So how can you make an intelligent decision with all this conflicting advice? Like Debbie, you'll probably want to seek out a second, even a third, opinion, from someone knowledgeable in the field.

Consulting with the Experts—Not an Easy Task

Does the following scenario have a familiar ring?

> *"On one side of the auditorium stage sat Profes-*
> *sor King, the chief of Ob/Gyn, a very big guy with*
> *a centurion voice. On the other side was Minnie*
> *Goldberg, who was about five feet tall and an en-*
> *docrinologist. King got up, with his residents in*
> *wide array, and said, 'Anybody who gives estro-*
> *gen to menopausal women is meddling with*

149

*nature.' There was a great 'Hurrah!' from his
side of the auditorium. Then Minnie got up and
said, 'Dr. King, anybody who would withhold estrogen from a menopausal woman is guilty of the
same crime as withholding insulin from a dia-
betic.' And there was tremendous clapping for her!"*
—ALFRED DASHE, M.D.,
recalling a debate about estrogens during his
residency in the late 1940s at the University of
California, San Francisco, Medical School

Although we know so much more about the female endocrine and reproductive systems now than we did 40 years ago,
the controversy still continues.

You're interested in what experts have to say on health
issues, so you read magazine and newspaper articles, and
maybe even studies in medical journals, that address your
questions regarding the pros and cons of HRT. As you have
probably already gathered, you won't necessarily get a con-
sensual opinion from all experts. And medical science has been
known to make mistakes. After estrogens were widely prescribed in the 1950s and 1960s to "keep women young forever," studies found an increased risk of endometrial cancer
from those large (by today's standards) and unopposed doses
of estrogens. Now hormone replacement therapy combines
about one-fourth of the earlier dosage of estrogen with a
progestin to protect against endometrial cancer. However,
experts are now divided about the effects of the progestins
added to the regimen. Some studies have noted that this form
of progesterone adversely affects the cholesterol level; and
there's complete disagreement about whether progestins prevent or cause breast cancer!

According to health-care advocates, this continued dis-agreement among experts is a danger sign for consumers. In testimony before the Senate Subcommittee on Aging's "Hear-ing on the Role of Menopause and Gender Differences in Aging on the Development of Disease in Mid-Life and Older Women" in April, 1991, Dr. Sidney M. Wolfe, Director of Public Citizen Health Research Group, quoted a University of Pennsylvania epidemiologist, Dr. Paul Stolley, in his caution to women: "The famous philosopher Bertrand Russell said that when the experts are not in agreement, the non-expert does well to suspend judgment. That could apply to HRT. The woman with a predictably high risk of developing osteoporosis might wish to run the known and unknown risks of HRT with careful monitoring for the fairly certain benefit in the preven-tion of osteoporosis; however, the woman with no special risk factors of osteoporosis would do well to consider waiting for a few years with the hope that new knowledge will permit a more informed choice."

An article in the September 1991 *Consumer Reports* entitled "The Estrogen Question," although generally favor-able about the use of HRT, conceded that "women who are facing menopause now need to decide what to do on the basis of less than perfect data."

"One of the problems with HRT," says Dr. Kaplan, "is that patients don't really see the day-to-day benefit—how it can prevent small, subtle vertebral fractures that lead to pain and discomfort as a woman gets older. But in terms of quality of life, how you feel, how strong your bones are, I think that affects people more than they realize."

The evidence for prevention of osteoporosis is compel-ling. No one wants to spend the last third of her life in pain and immobilized by repeated fractures or fear of them.

However, projecting into the future is always tricky business. Here are some steps you can begin to take now:

COMPILE A CHECKLIST OF YOUR OWN FAMILY AND PERSONAL HEALTH HISTORY. Table #1 at the end of the chapter is an example of the kind of information you and your physician will need to make the decision. In your own personal health and habits history, don't forget to include information about any past or present drug or alcohol abuse. Some of us may feel leery about discussing this with our doctors, but to make informed, intelligent decisions about health care, you and your physician need to have the whole picture.

START INTERVIEWING YOUR DOCTOR. What are his or her opinions about HRT and its usefulness or advisability in your case? Is your physician well versed in the problems of menopausal women? Is your physician willing to spend consultation time with you? Make yourself a partner in your health care. Most women see their gynecologists each year for pelvic exam and Pap smear. Dr. Kaplan thinks this is the ideal time to be discussing the issues of menopause.

"A good 50% of what I do as a reproductive endocrinologist [specialist in women's reproductive and infertility problems]," says Dr. Kaplan, "is just to talk with patients and explain things. My training makes me more interested in doing it. I think patients should demand this kind of time. I think patients should say, 'I would like to set up a 30-minute or a 45-minute appointment or whatever it takes so I can have my questions answered and expect to pay the physician for it.' That to me is the answer to all of this—that ev-

152

eryone needs to have an individual evaluation by somebody who can make sense of this for them."

DETERMINE IF YOU HAVE SPECIFIC AND REAL RISKS FOR OSTEOPOROSIS (see Table #2) *AND/OR HEART DISEASE* (see Table #3).

DETERMINE IF YOU HAVE DEFINITE CONTRAINDICATIONS FOR HRT. See Table #4, "Conditions that Definitely Contraindicate HRT," and Table #5, "Relative Risk Factors."

Do You Need Estrogens?

The estrogen decision must really be made on two levels: short-term and long-term. The reasons for each are summarized below. The risks of short-term HRT (two years or less) are relatively minor. Long-term HRT requires more assessment, although the screening your physician gives you for either should include the same tests (see Chapter Nine, "Commonsense Monitoring").

Short-Term HRT

From 75% to 80% of all menopausal women experience hot flashes. Of those women, 80% complain of them for more than one year and 25% to 50% for longer than five years. The intensity and severity differs from woman to woman. For Nancy, relief of menopausal symptoms would not be a compelling reason to begin taking hormones. But Freda, whose story you read about in Chapter Six, was nearly debilitated by hot flashes and sweating at night, along with severe mood swings and depression.

153

Nicky noted that vaginal dryness made intercourse quite uncomfortable for her. This is another indication for short-term HRT, in the form of either oral medication or a vaginal cream to moisten the vaginal tissues.

Long-Term HRT

According to the National Osteoporosis Foundation, osteoporosis, the bone-thinning disease, affects more than half of all women over 65. It's called the "silent thief" because until a fracture occurs, patients may not be aware they have the disease. Hormone replacement therapy is one of the main lines of defense against bone loss, although other drug therapies are currently being investigated.

The USC study of 8,881 postmenopausal women in Leisure World, near San Diego, showed an overall 20% reduced mortality rate in women who had ever used estrogens, and a 40% reduction in mortality in women currently using estrogens. Brian Henderson, M.D., and his co-researchers reported that most of this 40% reduction was due to fewer deaths from various types of heart and blood vessel disease. One large British study, which followed 4,544 long-term users of HRT and was reported in the *British Journal of Obstetrics and Gynecology,* also noted a beneficial effect of HRT on cardiovascular disease.

Should You Stay Away from Estrogens?

You may recall some of the risk factors for breast cancer from Chapter Four: no children or first children after 30, family history of breast cancer, and so on. While some physicians say a risk factor is reason enough to avoid estrogens, others will argue that women with strong risk factors can still be on HRT, with consistent and thorough monitoring. However, even if you have none of these risk factors, you should not assume you're free from risk of getting breast cancer. There is no way to predict the appearance and progress of this disease. Gloria Frankl, M.D., a radiologist and head of mammography at Kaiser Permanente's Sunset Center in Los Angeles, has kept records on 44,000 screenings done at her facility over the last 20 years. An astounding 34% of women who had detectable lumps shown in a mammogram had *none* of the risk factors present. Breast cancer is now more prevalent in our population than it was 20 years ago, and every woman should be diligent about getting periodic mammograms (the recommended schedule is in Chapter Nine, "Commonsense Monitoring") and supplementing those with monthly breast self-examinations (BSEs). By some statistics, most breast cancers are now 80% curable if they are caught early enough.

You and your doctor are the most qualified team for making the estrogen decision. Take time to really consider your options. By knowing your own benefit-risk ratio, you can make a more informed and rational decision. Once you make your decision, be assured that it's not cut in stone. If you experience difficulties on HRT, your doctor can make adjustments. If you decide not to begin HRT, remember that you can always change your mind later. Whatever your decision, you should not neglect your own checkups. To take the best care of yourself, you should always follow the practice of "Commonsense Monitoring," covered in the next chapter.

Table #1

PERSONAL AND FAMILY HEALTH HISTORY CHECKLIST

Question	Yes	No

Personal Health History:

1. Do you eat a balanced diet adequate in calcium (1,000 mg a day), as well as other essential vitamins and minerals?
2. Are you or have you ever been a heavy smoker?
3. Do you consume alcohol to excess? (More than two 12-oz. cans of beer, two 6-oz. glasses of wine, or 2 shots [1.5-oz. each] of whiskey or other hard liquor daily.)
4. Do you consume large amounts of caffeine? (Equivalent of a pot of coffee per day?)
5. Do you engage in weight-bearing exercise (walking, jogging, aerobics, weight training) for at least 20 minutes three times a week?

Do you have a history of:

1. Cardiovascular problems (heart attack, thrombophlebitis or embolism, coronary artery disease, cardiac edema, or hypertension?
2. Breast cancer?
3. Liver disease?
4. Insulin-dependent diabetes mellitus?
5. Diethylstilbestrol (DES) use during a pregnancy?
6. Gallbladder disease?
7. Uterine problems: endometrial cancer, fibroids, abnormal Pap smears, or undiagnosed abnormal bleeding?

Do your immediate family members—parents, siblings—have a history of:

1. Coronary artery disease?
2. DES use by your mother while pregnant with you?
3. Breast cancer?

Note: This list is not intended for diagnostic purposes, but you can bring it with you when you want to discuss HRT with your doctor.

156

Table #2

OSTEOPOROSIS—ARE YOU AT RISK?

Question	Yes	No
1. Do you have a small, thin frame, or are you Caucasian or Asian?		
2. Do you have a family history of osteoporosis?		
3. Are you a postmenopausal woman?		
4. Have you had an early or surgically induced menopause?		
5. Have you been taking excessive thyroid medication or high doses of cortisone-like drugs for asthma, arthritis, or cancer?		
6. Is your diet low in dairy products and other sources of calcium?		
7. Are you physically inactive?		
8. Do you smoke cigarettes or drink alcohol in excess?		

The more times you answer "yes," the greater your risk for developing osteoporosis.

Reprinted with permission from the National Osteoporosis Foundation, Washington, D.C., copyright 1991.

Table #3

RISK FACTORS FOR HEART DISEASE

Still the number one killer in America, heart and blood vessel diseases combined account for nearly 500,000 deaths (heart attack, stroke) of American women each year. Heart disease is not only a man's disease. Approximately half of all deaths due to heart disease each year are women. What are your chances of developing heart disease? Read the factors below to find out.

Unchangeable Risk Factors
• Age—the older you are, the more likely you are to get heart disease.
• Sex—after the menopause, women very quickly catch up to men, who are more at risk at younger ages.
• Race—African-Americans have higher average blood pressure levels, and are therefore at more risk for heart disease and stroke than Caucasians.
• Family history—If your immediate family members (parents, siblings) had or have heart disease, you are more likely to get it too.

Changeable Risk Factors
The following are risk factors which you can change, or for which your doctor can prescribe medications.
• Smoking—Nicotine and the other chemicals in cigarettes cause the blood vessels to constrict, which can exacerbate a problem with blood vessels that are already narrowed due to plaque buildup. Smoking also deprives your blood of oxygen by raising the level of carbon monoxide, and causes your heart rate to increase. If you smoke and want to quit, consult your local American Cancer Society or American Heart Association office for smoking cessation programs.
• High blood pressure—A reading of 140/90 (upper number is systolic pressure, the pressure of blood flow from your heart; lower number is diastolic, the measure of pressure between beats) is considered high. If you have high blood pressure, ask your physician what measures you can take to lower it. More than half of all women over age 55 have high blood pressure.

• Elevated cholesterol levels—A total blood cholesterol reading of between 200 and 239 is considered borderline and over 240 is high; HDL should be over 35 and LDL below 130 to be safe. If dietary and exercise measures don't work to lower your cholesterol levels, your physician may prescribe medication to lower them.

Source: American Heart Association, copyright 1989, "Silent Epidemic: The Truth About Women and Heart Disease."

Table #4

CONDITIONS THAT DEFINITELY CONTRAINDICATE HRT

The following diseases and conditions constitute risk factors that contraindicate HRT. Some conditions, such as undiagnosed uterine bleeding, may be removed as a contraindication if your doctor is able to identify and clear up the cause of the bleeding.

Liver disease (requires monitoring of serum estrogen)
Existing cardiovascular disease (of some types only)
History of gallbladder disease (not after gallbladder is removed, however)
Breast cancer
Endometrial cancer
History of thromboembolism
Undiagnosed uterine bleeding

Table #5

RELATIVE RISK FACTORS

The following conditions and risk factors constitute a relative risk for HRT. You and your physician will decide whether you might benefit from HRT even though you have such conditions. Of course, careful and regular monitoring is essential to ensure your continued health.

Family history of breast cancer
Insulin-dependent diabetes mellitus
Hypertension
Uterine fibroids or endometriosis
DES use—by you or your mother while pregnant with you

Table # 6

SHOULD YOU CONSIDER HORMONE REPLACEMENT THERAPY?

No	Maybe	Yes
Liver disease	Family history of breast cancer	Extreme discomfort with menopause (short-term)
Existing cardio-vascular disease	Diabetes mellitus	High risk for osteoporosis (long-term—20 years plus)
Breast cancer	Uterine fibroids or endometriosis	
Endometrial cancer	DES use	
Thromboembolism		Family history of heart disease before 55
Undiagnosed uterine bleeding		Other risk factors for coronary artery disease: high cholesterol, hypertension

9

Commonsense Monitoring

• • •

"My period stopped about four and a half months ago. I went in to see my doctor, because I wanted to make sure I wasn't pregnant. My doctor said I wasn't and that it must be menopause. She advised me to read up on estrogen and make my own decision about it. She didn't want to influence me, and she didn't really discuss it thoroughly. She just said, 'Read up on it.' I don't necessarily want to take estrogen, but my doctor claims it's safer now than it used to be—because of lower dosages—and that it prevents that terrible bone degenerating condition. I don't really like taking anything, *even aspirin. And I always think about the side effects associated with taking drugs. Besides, my mother never took estrogen, and she's okay."*

—SUSAN, age 49

Susan is only beginning to inform herself about the pros and cons of estrogen. By the time you reach menopause, it's more than likely that your doctor will also raise the question. He or she may supply more information than Susan's did, but the decision will remain in your hands.

"I think it's essential for the patient to remain informed. That's a message of modern medicine, that patients have to take a great deal of responsibility for their own bodies. This is a subject that requires seeking out knowledge, and if their physicians can't provide it, they'd better get a new one."
—LEON SPEROFF, M.D.,
reproductive endocrinologist,
Oregon Health Sciences University, Portland

You may feel overwhelmed by the amount of information required to come to a conclusion about estrogen. Aside from available published material and the information your physician can provide, consulting with friends and family members may also help you with your decision. And there's your own body and the information you can get from common-sense monitoring. Blood tests, physical exams, and hip X-rays won't give you the entire picture or all the answers. But if you are attentive, have the right doctor, and get the right tests, you'll have adequate information upon which to base your health-care choices.

Even if you do decide to start hormone replacement therapy, your decision need not be a final one. Although some of the women I talked to have been taking estrogen or estrogen/progestin replacement for 7, 10, even 20 years without problems, others have been experiencing troubling side effects. Nicky's unexplained and unusually heavy bleeding, for instance, is still cause for concern for her and her doctor.

Sophia, who decided at menopause not to take estrogen, has now reversed that decision. Development of kidney stones made it impossible for her to continue large doses of calcium, and a subsequent hip X-ray revealed that she had osteoporosis. So she agreed to start on HRT to retard the disease.

Each woman brings her own unique health history to this question. You may not fit any of the standard profiles for those who should or should not take HRT. That's why it's critical to have a physician who will treat you as an individual. During this process, self-monitoring, along with regular checkups, can be a real ally.

By the time you've reached the age of 40, you should already be familiar with regular health-care screening tests: a baseline mammogram, regular blood tests, pelvic exams, Pap smears, and breast exams. When you begin to enter menopause, it's a good idea to monitor your own symptoms by jotting them down in a notebook. Keeping track of when you had your last period—as Susan did—will help you and your doctor determine when you are truly menopausal and when to either consider HRT or rule it out in favor of alternative therapies.

Once made, your estrogen decision will most probably offer continuing choices, even challenges. If you decide to begin HRT and experience uncomfortable or alarming side effects, your doctor will have to assess what additional tests may be necessary, alter dosages, or decide whether you should discontinue.

As with all other aspects surrounding the estrogen decision, you should discuss with your physician how he or she will monitor your health while you're on hormones. There are differences of opinion regarding which tests should be given, and how often. "To prescribe hormone replacement therapy and then add the statement, 'I'll see you next year,' is out of the question," points out Sonia Hamburger, clinical instructor at UCSD's Menopause Clinic in La Jolla, California.

Depending on your individual health history, it may be advisable for you to have checkups more often than once a year. For instance, if you have a family history of high blood cholesterol levels (hypercholesterolemia), your physician may recommend, along with your treatment regimen, that you have your cholesterol levels evaluated every six months.

In this chapter, you'll learn about the usual tests and evaluations that doctors perform before and during HRT. How extensive these tests are will depend on your health history and to some extent on what your doctor feels is necessary, as well as on what kind of health plan you have. Knowing which tests are available can help you make pertinent decisions about whether you're with the right doctor, or the right health plan.

You may have some homework to do. Unfortunately, our health-care delivery system isn't set up to encourage physicians to spend much time on prevention and health education. Third-party payors (insurance companies), health maintenance organizations (HMOs) and preferred provider organizations (PPOs) are very conscious of cost containment, sometimes to the detriment of pursuing all diagnostic avenues. Physicians are reimbursed for procedures they perform, and the payors have strict rules about what is "customary and reasonable."

"The problem is that the medical profession doesn't get paid for telling people how to change their eating habits or exercise regimen, or how to deal with symptomatology or even smoking cessation, so there's very little emphasis on this type of approach. I think that's a big, big mistake," says Lewis Kuller, an epidemiologist at the University of Pittsburgh. In an ideal world, according to Dr. Kuller, all physicians would function like pediatricians, whose function is primarily prevention. So, in this imperfect world and imperfect health-care system, you have to learn how to work the system. Part of that involves knowing what's available and what's standard according to the experts. You may have to be prepared to justify certain tests to an insurance company, pay a percentage of the cost yourself, or pay out of pocket for a second opinion.

Tests Before HRT

Some physicians gauge a woman's menopausal status solely by the clinical symptoms she presents—hot flashes, infrequent or absent menstrual periods, drying vagina, and so forth. However, most physicians will also order blood tests to confirm that you are indeed going through menopause. One of the most common tests measures the level of FSH (follicle stimulating hormone). The ovaries usually respond to FSH by releasing a mature ovum. When the ovaries don't respond, the hypothalamus and pituitary step up the release of FSH and LH (luteinizing hormone) to nudge the ovaries into action. An elevated FSH level confirms that the brain is trying hard to force the ovary to make estrogen. If the estrogen level in the blood is low, this confirms that menopause is the problem.

Another way to confirm that you are in menopause is for your doctor to take a sampling of your vaginal epithelial cells, which can be analyzed for the effect of estrogen. Internist Alfred Dashe evaluates the estrogen level on a Pap smear according to the maturation index. If a patient has adequate estrogen, he does not suggest HRT unless the woman is also experiencing hot flashes.

Dr. Dashe points out that a woman can exhibit adequate estrogen effect from the Pap smear reading and still have terrible hot flashes. If your hot flashes, the most common menopausal symptom, are frequent and exceedingly uncomfortable, HRT will give you relief. Again, the most common tests for establishing that you are in menopause:

- Observation of clinical symptoms—infrequent or disappearing menstrual periods, hot flashes, vaginal dryness and thinning
- FSH and estrogen levels in the blood
- Vaginal smears

Evaluation for HRT

If you and your doctor agree to proceed with hormone replacement therapy, you must be thoroughly evaluated first. If the prescribing physician has not been your primary doctor, he or she should take a complete medical history. This will include your past medical records and family health history (see Chapter Eight for lists of family health risks), your reports of menopausal symptoms (hot flushes, infrequent or discontinued menstruation, pain upon intercourse, changes in sexual desire, urinary urgency or incontinence, night sweats, mood changes, insomnia, fatigue, headaches), any medications you are currently using, and any conditions for which you are presently being treated. In addition, the other screenings that should be performed include:

- A gynecological exam, which, if you're menopausal, may reveal: sparse pubic hair, pale and thin vaginal lining, a cervix that may be flush with the vagina instead of protruding into it, a smaller uterus, and ovaries that are not palpable.

- Urinalysis

- Blood pressure

- Complete blood count

- Fasting blood sugars

- Cholesterol (including total cholesterol, as well as HDL and LDL) and triglyceride levels

- Liver function tests

- Thyroid function

- Pap smear, including a maturation index. (If this index shows that most of the cells present are parabasal cells, this will reveal minimal or no estrogen effect.)

- Mammogram—this should be compared with your baseline. More on mammography later in the chapter.

Tests Not Universally Performed (but suggested if you are under specific risk)

- Bone density study. This test is performed by intravenously injecting an isotopic dye and then taking an x-ray (which takes only about 5 to 10 minutes) called a dual photon absorptiometry (DPA). The reading given on your hip will be compared with the average readings for someone your age. If you are at risk for osteoporosis, your physician may recommend this test. And if you're in doubt about starting HRT, you may want to consider having a DPA. However, this is still not reimbursable by most insurance companies, and can cost from $75 to $300.

- Additional blood work for clotting factors, which estrogen can also affect. This would depend on your medical history—specifically, if you have a family history of thromboembolism (formation of blood clots).

- Endometrial biopsy, performed by taking a scraping from the uterine lining, is similar to a D&C. Like a D&C, it can be done in a doctor's office. It causes some discomfort but is warranted when a woman has recently experienced abnormal and unexplained bleeding. By examining the tissue taken, the presence of hyperplastic or cancerous cells can be picked up or a diagnosis such as uterine fibroids or endometriosis made. If a woman has an intact uterus and is taking or is considering taking unopposed estrogens, she may be a candidate for the biopsy since unopposed estrogens have been linked to endometrial cancer. Taking estrogen and progestin in combination still doesn't get you out of the woods entirely, however. Dr. R. Don Gambrell, Jr., of the Medical College of Georgia, reports that he rarely performs biopsies on women taking estrogen and progestin except for those who develop unexplained bleeding (not the monthly withdrawal bleeding precipitated by the progestin).

- A progesterone challenge test entails taking 10 mg Provera for 5 to 10 days. If no bleeding occurs, the endometrial biopsy is not usually necessary. However, if there is bleeding in response to the progesterone challenge, an endometrial biopsy will usually follow.

- Pelvic ultrasound is a noninvasive test, performed in a radiologist's office, that can be used to assess the thickness of the uterine cavity. Some physicians are leaning toward using this test instead of a biopsy, or as a supplement to the endometrial biopsy, to evaluate buildup of the uterine lining.

Regular Screenings While on HRT

If you're in good health and have had no serious illness, you may only need the basic follow-up tests. These are performed annually and semiannually:

Annual Tests

- Pap smear, if you have an intact uterus
- Mammogram, if you're over 50 (may be required after 40 for women with specific risk factors). Current American Cancer Society guidelines for mammography recommend screenings for women between 40 and 49 every one or two years.
- Pelvic and rectal exam

Semiannual Tests

- Blood pressure reading
- Hemoglobin (red blood cell count)
- Clinical breast examination by the physician
- Urinalysis

What if You Have Problems?

Taking hormones is serious business. It's imperative for you to report any unexpected or unusually heavy bleeding to your doctor. When you begin HRT, ask your doctor what is normal and what you should be alert to. If you have a lot of bleeding and if it occurs other than during the expected, monthly withdrawal bleeding caused by the progestins, your physician may decide to perform the progesterone challenge test. If bleeding occurs, an endometrial biopsy may be necessary.

Even though HRT has not been positively shown to cause gallstones, it could happen. You should alert your doctor if you have these symptoms: indigestion, belching, occasional nausea, and pain in your upper right abdomen.

Pay attention to any new breast lumps or breast changes. The following section discusses mammograms and monthly breast self-examination (BSE).

Self-Monitoring

- Schedule a mammogram appointment. Don't wait for your physician to remind you. Know how often you should be getting one, by following the guidelines recommended by the American Cancer Society:

- Obtain a baseline mammogram sometime between the ages of 35 and 39—perhaps sooner, if you have family members with breast cancer. A baseline will give your radiologists something with which to compare future mammograms of your breasts.

  If you are moving out of the area, be sure to take your baseline and subsequent mammographies with you. A new baseline may not be as reliable.

  Clinical instructor Sonia Hamburger of UCSD's Menopause Clinic urges women to have their mammograms read on the spot, so there won't be any suspense about the results. However, if you're a member of an HMO, such as Kaiser, this may not always be possible, since they usually notify you of your mammogram results by mail.

  Make sure the equipment being used is *dedicated*—that is, used for mammographies and nothing else. You can also check with the facility to make sure they're accredited by the American College of Radiology and that their equipment is calibrated (the levels of radiation tested for leakage and proper low levels—no more than 200 milliRads per study) on a regular basis.

- Between the ages of 40 and 49, have a mammogram done every one to two years.

- Over the age of 50, have a mammogram every year.

Doing a Monthly BSE

Monthly breast self-examination should be a part of every woman's health-care regimen. Radiologist and mammography specialist Gloria Frankl, M.D., of Kaiser Permanente in Los Angeles, emphasizes that BSE is not a substitute for mammography and regular clinical examinations by your doctor—it should be a *supplement.* Mammography can detect a lump so small that it is "occult," or "discreet," not felt by palpating the breast. It can also detect lumps that can't be felt because they're deeper. If you do feel a lump during your BSE, visit your doctor. Not every lump is cancerous, but you need to follow up on any new lumps or breast changes by seeking medical attention. The earlier you catch a cancer, the better your chances for cure.

The methods of doing BSE have been refined over the years. You may want to look at the diagrams on the next pages to familiarize yourself with the process, which is very thorough. If you know you have fibrocystic breasts, it's a good idea to draw a pencil diagram of where the benign masses in your breasts are. That way, you can refer to the "map" when you do your BSE to see if there have been changes.

Clinical Breast Exams

In addition, your doctor should do a breast exam when you visit for your six-month and/or yearly checkups. Physicians are often more experienced in palpating (feeling) for lumps. The American Cancer Society also recommends that you practice your BSE techniques while your doctor or nurse practitioner watches. If you are doing the procedure incorrectly, they can offer tips on correct technique.

Commonsense monitoring doesn't come with absolute guarantees. However, it's one way to take charge of your health and participate as a full partner in your own health care. The more you know about your own body, the better able you'll be to make informed, intelligent choices.

Breast Self-Examination:

A NEW APPROACH All women over 20 should practice monthly breast self-examination (BSE). Regular and complete BSE can help you find changes in your breasts that occur between clinical breast examinations (by a health professional) and mammograms.

Women should examine their breasts when they are least tender, usually seven days after the start of the menstrual period. Women who have entered menopause or are pregnant or breastfeeding, and women who have silicone implants, should continue to examine their breasts once a month. Breastfeeding mothers should examine their breasts when all milk has been expressed.

If a woman discovers a lump or detects any changes, she should seek medical attention. Nine out of ten women will not develop breast cancer and most breast changes are *not* cancerous.

HOW TO DO BSE

1. Lie down and put a pillow under your right shoulder. Place your right arm behind your head.
2. Use the finger pads of the three middle fingers on your left hand to feel for lumps or thickening. Your finger pads are the top third of each finger.

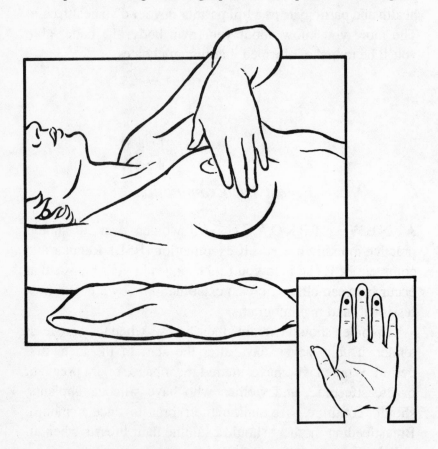

3. Press hard enough to know how your breast feels. If you're not sure how hard to press, ask your health care provider. Or try to copy the way your health care provider uses the finger pads during a breast exam. Learn what your breast feels like most of the time. A firm ridge in the lower curve of each breast is normal.

4. Move around the breast in a set way. You can choose the circle (A), the up and down line (B), or the wedge (C). Do it the same way every time. It will help you to make sure that you've gone over the entire breast area, and to remember how your breast feels each month.

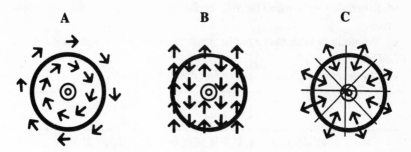

A B C

5. Now examine your left breast using right hand finger pads.

You might want to check your breasts while standing in front of a mirror right after you do your BSE each month. You might also want to do an extra BSE while you're in the shower. Your soapy hands will glide over the wet skin making it easy to check how your breasts feel.

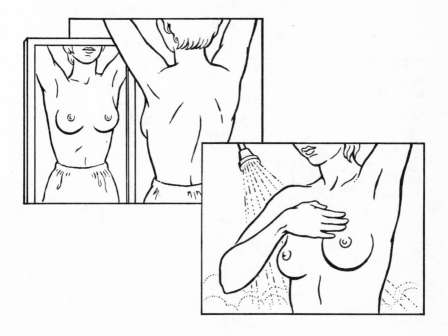

175

PLAN OF ACTION

Every woman should have a personal breast health plan of action:

✔ Discuss the American Cancer Society breast cancer detection guidelines with your health-care professional.

✔ Schedule your clinical breast examination and mammogram as appropriate.

✔ Do monthly BSE. Ask your health professional for feedback on your BSE skills.

✔ Report any changes to your health-care professional.

AMERICAN CANCER SOCIETY GUIDELINES FOR BREAST CANCER DETECTION

Breast Self-Examination:	Age 20 and over: monthly
Clinical Breast Examination:	Age 20–39: every 3 years
	Age 40 and over: yearly
Mammography:	Age 35–39: Baseline
	Age 40–49: every 1–2 years
	Age 50 and over: yearly

The American Cancer Society. By permission.
Revised 12/88
6438.39

Conclusion—
The Balanced
Approach

• • •

Most women looking ahead to menopause want to know: Should I take estrogens? There is no simple yes or no answer to that question, as I found out by talking with dozens of physicians, researchers, and health-care advocates across the country.

In about seven years, I'm going to be in the same boat as the women I talked with. Unless the mainstream medical community's thinking changes radically by then, my own doctor will likely suggest hormone replacement therapy.

How will I respond when she asks, "Have you thought about taking estrogens?" I decided to write this book because I was looking for a balanced approach to the estrogen question. I don't want *my* decision made for me and I don't want it to be made by default. I want to have enough information to discuss my decision intelligently and thoroughly.

The majority of gynecologists and reproductive endocrinologists I interviewed are in favor of HRT, both for short-term treatment of menopausal symptoms and because of its long-term benefits for a woman's health and quality—even quantity—of life.

Those opposing long-term HRT sound just as convincing. But the pendulum has been swinging back and forth for some time about long-term HRT. If you believe Sidney M. Wolfe, M.D., director of Public Citizen Health Research Group, "a lot of the enthusiasm [for large-scale use of HRT] is funded by Wyeth-Ayerst and American Home Products, who manufacture Premarin. . . . HRT has been heavily promoted," says Wolfe. "And a lot of these people are not able to sort out the myths from the realities. The problem is that sometimes physicians don't take the time or, in some cases, have the understanding to sort all this out, and they succumb to the pressure both from the company directly and indirectly through their peers who get paid to give pep talks [about the hormones]."

Lewis Kuller, a University of Pittsburgh epidemiologist, thinks the enthusiasm for HRT is more complicated than this. "Part of the enthusiasm," he says, "is the fact that people have done studies that show it reduces the risk of osteoporosis. Estrogen has always been popular because it does relieve [menopausal] symptoms. And that's important. The problem is that [the indication for HRT] has become lesser and lesser. A woman has three hot flashes and suddenly decides, 'Hey, I better take estrogen therapy.' I know women who go to a doctor and the doctor says, '*All* women should be on estrogen therapy.' That's dreadful and that's wrong."

According to R. Don Gambrell, Jr., M.D., a researcher who is also in private practice, it's the epidemiologists who are creating the problem. He attended a September 1991 meeting in London along with 13 epidemiologists and reports their 20-year frustration at not being able to prove that estrogens increase the risk of breast cancer.

"As the only clinician on the program, I suggested to them that enough is enough—quit scaring our patients with basically negative reports. The Swedish study (published in 1989 in the *New England Journal of Medicine*) caused thousands of women to go off their hormone therapy even though it has since been totally refuted."

While the experts go to battle over the advisability of estrogen therapy, as they have since the late 1940s, what should we as women be doing?

We should be carefully considering our own individual options. You do not have to take female hormones—there are alternatives. By the same token, if you decide to try HRT, you're entitled to have ongoing medical consultation during every critical juncture. The common theme to the estrogen decision, repeated by both doctors and patients, is that the decision and the therapy must have an individualized approach. Says Dr. Cynthia A. Stuenkel, reproductive endocrinologist and Associate Professor of Reproductive Medicine at the University of California, San Diego Medical School, "I like my patients to say, 'She recommended it and we agreed,' rather than, 'My doctor put me on hormones.'"

There is no doubt that HRT is beneficial, even needed, for some women. By ruling it out arbitrarily because it's "unnatural," you may be robbing yourself of a chance to significantly improve the quality of the last 30 years of your life. Like many of the women I interviewed, I don't like taking medications. A multivitamin and occasional Tylenol for a very bad headache are about it. But is this a valid enough reason *not* to consider HRT?

My research for this book has allowed me to compare my own risk factors with the standard profiles. My father died in his early 50s of acute myocardial infarction (heart attack). And each year 250,000 American women over the age of 55 die of heart attacks. This is a risk factor I can personally relate to. Even though some researchers still disagree about estrogen's benefit to the heart, larger population studies, such as the

Leisure World study, have demonstrated that women taking estrogen have fewer heart attacks and live longer than those who don't take estrogens. That's a very compelling reason for me to consider HRT.

As Lewis Kuller points out, there are plenty of alternatives for lowering your risk of heart disease: You can lose weight, exercise, and monitor your cholesterol levels regularly. But simply "doing the right thing" is not a guarantee that we'll stay well. So in my case HRT may help provide that guarantee.

The estrogen decision is a serious one, but it doesn't have to be rushed. We have time to carefully consider our own individual plan of action. As national attention becomes more focused on women's health issues, the data will continue to mount. Time is on our side.

Conventional wisdom has it that women are, by nature or by conditioning, caretakers. This can sometimes mean that we put off taking care of our own needs until those of our family and friends are met. Most of us have at some time or another put off going to the doctor. Unless we're in pain or have a clear symptom it's often easy to postpone regular checkups.

I want the years after menopause to be as productive and full as possible. And with the right decisions, they can be. Menopause can be a great opportunity to take better care of ourselves. As we enter midlife, we can take an active role in examining our health and lifestyle choices, and thinking about what we'd like to change and improve. The first step is acquiring sufficient knowledge to make our own informed estrogen decision.

List of Resources

The following organizations make available information on menopause, hormone replacement and related topics, usually for a nominal fee.

National Women's Health Network
1325 G Street, N.W.
Washington, D.C. 20005
(202) 347-1140

Information packets are available for $10. Information on specific topics available for an additional $5; or you may join the organization for $25.

National Osteoporosis Foundation
1625 Eye Street, N.W., No. 822
Washington, D.C. 20006
(202) 223-2226

Information in the form of pamphlets, photocopied research studies and more is available.

North American Menopause Society (NAMS)
c/o Cleveland Menopause Clinic
29001 Cedar Road, No. 600
Cleveland, OH 44124

The Society holds an annual conference at various locations throughout the U.S. and Canada. You are invited to join NAMS for $25 and receive mailings and information.

American College of Obstetricians and Gynecologists
409 12th Street, S.W.
Washington, D.C. 20024-2188
(202) 638-5577

ACOG publishes a large variety of pamphlets and brochures
on specific gynecological problems and conditions.

Glossary

· · ·

Abstract A summary or abridgment of an article, book, research study, etc.

Adaptogenic herbs Herbs that stimulate the body's immune system to encourage self-regulation.

Amenorrhea Absence or abnormal cessation of menstruation for at least three months in a woman with prior menses.

Androgen Male hormone.

Anovulatory cycles Times when an egg is not released from the ovaries.

Arthralgia Joint pain.

Aspirate To draw in or out by suction.

Atresia Degeneration.

Bone density study Sophisticated, noninvasive X-rays done of the hip, performed by intravenously injecting an isotopic dye and then taking an X-ray called a dual photon absorptiometry (DPA). *See* dual photon absorptiometry.

Bone remodeling A process that takes place continuously inside the bone marrow, where large multinuclear cells (osteoclasts) break down old bone cells (resorption). Then new bone is formed and the cycle repeats.

Breast self-examination (BSE) A technique that enables a woman to detect any changes in her breasts, useful in the early detection of breast cancer. BSE should be done once a month soon after the completion of the menstrual period, when the breasts are not tender, and on a monthly basis after menopause.

Catecholamines Biologically active amines, epinephrine and norepinephrine, derived from the amino acid tyrosine. They affect the nervous and cardiovascular systems, metabolic rate, temperature, and smooth muscle.

Climacteric The period from perimenopause to cessation of menopausal symptoms. From the Greek *klimakter*, "a rung of the ladder."

Conjugated estrogens Combined estrogens from the urine of pregnant mares. Contained in one of the most widely prescribed oral estrogens, Premarin.

Corpus luteum A yellowish mass or casing that forms around the mature graafian follicle containing the egg; it secretes estrogen and progesterone. *See* luteinizing hormone.

Diastolic pressure In blood pressure readings, the lower number, which measures the pressure between beats. *See* systolic pressure.

Diethylstilbestrol (DES) A synthetic preparation possessing estrogenic properties. It has been found to be related to subsequent vaginal malignancies in the daughters of mothers who received it during pregnancy.

Dilatation and curettage (D&C) A procedure during which the cervix is dilated and the uterine wall is scraped.

Dong quai An adaptogenic herb that contains phyto-estrogens (plant estrogens), used in the Orient to treat hot flashes, anxiety, depression, and insomnia. *See* adaptogenic herbs.

184

Double-blind study A study in which neither researchers nor participants know which volunteers are taking the drug being studied or the placebo. *See* placebo.

Dual photon absorptiometry (DPA) A special kind of X-ray using two beams of light to measure the density of bone, typically the hip or forearm.

Dyspareunia Difficult or painful intercourse.

Embolism Sudden blocking of an artery by a clot.

Endogenous estrogen Estrogen originating within the body, made in the adrenal gland, ovaries, and fatty tissues.

Endometrial biopsy Excision of a small piece of uterine tissue for microscopic examination.

Endometrium Lining of the uterus.

Epidemiologists Scientists who study factors that cause and influence the incidence and distribution of disease in entire populations.

Estradiol The most potent of three estrogen compounds made in the body. Produced by the ovary, it is part of the complicated feedback system between the hypothalamus, pituitary, and ovary that results in the normal monthly ovulatory cycle.

Estriol A relatively weak estrogen compound, produced as a by-product of estradiol and estrone metabolism.

Estrogen receptor-positive Able to bind with and be affected by estrogen; most critical in determining whether a cancerous tumor is affected by estrogen.

Estrone A low-level estrogen compound converted from androgens in fatty tissue.

Estropipate A synthetic estrogen.

Exogenous estrogen Estrogen that has been developed outside the body, either synthetically or biologically.

Fibrocystic disease A benign condition of the breasts in which clumps of tissue occasionally produce noncancerous lumps.

Follicle stimulating hormone (FSH) A hormone secreted by the pituitary that stimulates the ovaries.

Ginseng A Chinese herb sometimes used by naturopathic physicians to treat menopausal symptoms, such as hot flashes.

Gonadotropins Hormones, such as FSH and LH (luteinizing hormone), that stimulate the ovaries. *See* follicle stimulating hormone *and* luteinizing hormone.

Graafian follicle A mature follicle of the ovary. Beginning with puberty and continuing until menopause, except during pregnancy, a graafian follicle develops at approximately monthly intervals. Each follicle contains a nearly mature ovum which, when it ruptures, is discharged from the ovary, a process called ovulation. *See* ovulation.

High-density lipoprotein (HDL) The "good" cholesterol.

Hormone replacement therapy (HRT) A monthly regimen of estrogen and progestin given to offset the effects of lowered estrogen levels in postmenopausal women.

Hot flash Also called hot flush. A sudden, inappropriate excitation of heat-release mechanisms, causing skin on the face and upper torso to flush, accompanied by various degrees of sweating.

Hypercholesterolemia Excessive amount of cholesterol in the blood.

Hyperplasia An abnormal growth of cells, sometimes indicating a precancerous condition.

Hyperthyroidism A condition caused by excessive secretion of the thyroid glands, which increases the basal metabolic rate, causing an increased demand for food to support this metabolic activity.

Hysterectomy Surgical removal of the uterus. Removal of the uterus alone is usually called partial hysterectomy; removal of uterus and ovaries is called complete hysterectomy.

Kegel exercises Exercises for strengthening the perineal muscles (between the vagina and anus) of the female.

Low-density lipoprotein (LDL) The "bad" cholesterol. *See* high-density lipoprotein.

Luteinizing hormone (LH) Hormone secreted by the pituitary that stimulates release of the ovum from the graafian follicle, resulting in ovulation. *See* corpus luteum.

Menarche The onset of menses.

Menopause That period which marks the permanent cessation of menstrual activity.

Myocardial infarction Heart attack.

Naturopath One who practices a therapeutic system that does not rely on drugs or standard medical therapy but may employ nonpharmacological methods such as acupuncture and herbs, based on Oriental theories of healing, or homeopathic or chiropractic methods.

Nulliparous Never having borne a child.

Oophorectomy Removal of the ovaries only. Sometimes also called female castration.

Osteoclasts   Large multinuclear cells that play a major role in bone remodeling, breaking down old bone before new bone is formed.

Osteopenia   Loss of bone mass.

Osteoporosis   The "brittle bones" disease; increased porosity of the bones.

Ovulation   The periodic ripening and rupture of the mature graafian follicle and the discharge of the ovum from the ovary's cortex. Ovulation occurs approximately 14 days before the next menstrual period. *See* graafian follicle.

Perimenopause   The time around, or just prior to, menopause.

Phytogens   Plant estrogens.

Placebo   Inactive substance used in controlled studies of drugs. The placebo is given to a group of patients and the drug being tested is given to a similar group; then the results obtained in the two groups are compared. *See* double-blind study.

Primiparity   The first full-term pregnancy.

Progesterone challenge test   Diagnostic test in which progesterone is given orally for a period of days. When the hormone is stopped, the physician looks for the absence or presence of uterine bleeding, then makes a determination of possible disease based on the results.

Progestin   Synthetic progesterone.

Prophylactic   A preventive measure.

Rapid eye movement (REM)   Cyclic movement of the closed eyes during sleep. Often referred to as "deep sleep," this period of sleep is strongly associated with dreaming. Decreased estrogen levels during menopause are thought to interfere with REM sleep.

Remodeling   In the bone, the process of breaking down and renewal of bone tissue. *See* bone remodeling.

Reproductive endocrinologist   A subspecialty in the field of gynecology that requires additional training and board certification.

Retinal thrombosis   A blood clot in the eye vessels.

Resorption   The dissolution and assimilation of tissue.

Stress incontinence   Inability to prevent escape of urine during stress such as laughing, coughing, or sneezing. A common consequence of vaginal delivery and aging.

Surgical menopause   Complete hysterectomy or oophorectomy—removal of the ovaries only. *See* hysterectomy.

Systolic pressure   In blood pressure readings, the upper number, which measures the pressure of blood flow from the heart. *See* diastolic pressure.

Thrombophlebitis   Blood clots in the vein.

Unopposed estrogens   Oral or injectable estrogen without the addition of progesterone.

Vaginal atrophy   A dryness and thinning of the vaginal wall.

Vaginitis   Inflammation of the vagina.

Weight-bearing exercise   Exercise in which a load is placed on the skeleton through a high- or low-impact aerobics routine, walking, or lifting weights.

Notes

. . .

INTRODUCTION

1. Jerome Abrams, M.D., M.P.H., "Estrogen Replacement for the 1990s," *New Jersey Medicine* 88 (March 1991): 177–179.

2. Sidney M. Wolfe, M.D., and Rhoda Donkin Jones, "Hormone Replacement Therapy," in *Women's Health Alert* (Reading, MA: Addison-Wesley Publishing Company, Inc., 1991): 194.

3. Leon Speroff, M.D., Robert H. Glass, M.D., and Nathan Kase, M.D., "The Ovary from Conception to Senescence," in *Clinical Gynecologic Endocrinology and Infertility,* Fourth Ed. (Baltimore: Williams & Wilkins, 1989): 122–126, 135.

4. Lori Miller Kase, "The Mythology of Menopause," *Health* (March 1991): 80–95.

5. Greg Spencer, Department of Projections, U.S. Census Bureau; April 1992 interview.

6. Speroff et al., op. cit., 137–146.

7. *Physicians' Desk Reference,* 46th Ed. (Montvale, New Jersey: Medical Economics Data, 1992): 2510, 2356.

8. "The Estrogen Question," *Consumer Reports,* September 1991: 587.

9. R. Don Gambrell, Jr., M.D., "The Menopause," "State of the Art in Medicine," *Investigative Radiology* 21 (April 1986): 369–377.

10. "The Estrogen Question," op. cit., 590.

11. Judith Sachs, *What Women Should Know About Menopause* (New York: Dell Publishing, 1991).

CHAPTER ONE

1. Speroff, op. cit., 134–135.

2. Greg Spencer, Department of Projections, U.S. Census Bureau.

3. The Postmenopausal Estrogen/Progestin Interventions (PEPI) Background, Department of Health and Human Services, October 1991.

4. Lila E. Nachtigall and Joan Rattner Heilman, "Is Estrogen Safe?" in *Estrogen: The Facts Can Change Your Life* (New York: HarperCollins, 1991): 22–25.

5. C. Donnell Turner, Ph.D., and Joseph T. Bagnara, Ph.D., "Endocrinology of the Ovary," in *General Endocrinology,* Sixth Ed., (Philadelphia: W. B. Saunders Co., 1981): 456–469.

6. Peter O. Kohler, M.D., and Richard M. Jordan, M.D., Eds., "The Normal Ovary," in *Clinical Endocrinology* (New York: John Wiley & Sons, 1986): 312–314.

7. Thurman Gillespy, III, M.D., and Marjorie P. Gillespy, M.D., "Osteoporosis," "Metabolic Bone Disease," *Radiologic Clinics of North America* 29 (January 1991): 77–78.

8. Overview: HHS and Private Sector Efforts in Osteoporosis, Department of Health and Human Services, National Institute of Arthritis and Musculoskeletal and Skin Diseases, 1991, 1–7.

9. "Estrogen Replacement Therapy," *Mayo Clinic Letter* (May 1991): 7.

10. Speroff, op. cit., 67–68.

11. *Dorland's Illustrated Medical Dictionary,* 27th Ed. (Philadelphia: W. B. Saunders Co., 1988): 584.

12. Speroff, op. cit., 129.

13. Janet Zand, N.D., O.M.D., "Menopause, A Comfortable Transition," *Delicious!* (November/December 1991): 35–36.

14. John A. McLachlan, Ed., *Estrogens in the Environment,* Proceedings of the Symposium on Estrogens in the Environment, Raleigh, South Carolina, September 1979.

15. Speroff, op. cit., 122–130.

16. Kohler, op. cit., 313.

17. Constance R. Martin, Ph.D., "The Female Reproductive System," in *Endocrine Physiology* (New York: Oxford University Press, 1985): 671–672.

18. Francis S. Greenspan, M.D., Ed., "Disorders of the Ovary and Female Reproductive Tract," in *Basic and Clinical Endocrinology* (Norwalk, Connecticut: Appleton & Lange, 1985): 249.

19. Maureen Dalton, "The Menopause," in *Gynaecological Endocrinology: A Guide to Understanding and Management* (Oradell, New Jersey: Medical Economics Books, 1989): 117.

CHAPTER TWO

1. "Estrogen Replacement Therapy," *American College of Obstetrics and Gynecology Technical Bulletin* 93 (June 1986).

2. James W. Long, M.D., *The Essential Guide to Prescription Drugs* (New York: HarperCollins, 1992): 489–494, 654–657.

3. Virginia Burke Karb, R.N., M.S.N., Sherry F. Queener, Ph.D., and Julia B. Freeman, Ph.D., Eds., *Handbook of Drugs for Nursing Practice* (St. Louis: The C. V. Mosby Company, 1989): 625–636.

4. R. Don Gambrell, Jr., M.D., *Estrogen Replacement Therapy User Guide* (Dallas: Essential Medical Information Systems, Inc., 1989).

5. Speroff, op. cit., 150–155.

6. Nachtigall, op. cit., 158–189.

7. *Physicians' Desk Reference,* op. cit.

8. Thrifty and Sav-On pharmacies, Los Angeles, California.

9. Roslyn B. Alfin-Slater, Ph.D., "How Medicines Affect Your Nutrient Reserves," *UCLA Health Insights* 3 (February 1985): 3–4.

10. "Transdermal Estradiol: A Review," *Drugs* 40, No. 4, 1990, 579.

11. P. R. Clisham et al., "Long-Term Transdermal Estradiol Therapy: Effects on Endometrial Histology and Bleeding Patterns," *Obstetrics and Gynecology* 79 (February 1992): 196–201.

12. "Estrogen Use," American College of Obstetrics and Gynecology Patient Education pamphlet #APO66, May 1986.

CHAPTER THREE

1. "Osteoporosis: Cause, Treatment, Prevention," National Institute of Arthritis and Musculoskeletal and Skin Diseases, National Institutes of Health, NIH Publication 86-2226, Revised May 1986.

2. "The Menopause Time of Life," National Institute on Aging, NIH Publication 86-2461, Revised July 1986.

3. Speroff, op. cit., 137–146.

4. "Should You Take Estrogen?" Age Page, National Institute on Aging, NIH fact sheet, U.S. Department of Health and Human Services, 1988, 195–194.

5. Jerome Abrams, M.D., M.P.H., "Estrogen Replacement for the 1990s," *New Jersey Medicine* 88 (March 1991): 177–179.

6. Edward G. Lufkin et al., "Estrogen Replacement Therapy: Current Recommendations," *Mayo Clinic Proceedings* 63 (1988): 453–460.

7. Deborah A. Metzger, M.D., Ph.D., and Charles B. Hammond, M.D., "Are Estrogens Indicated for the Treatment of Postmenopausal Women?" *Drug Intelligence and Clinical Pharmacy* 22 (June 1988): 493–496.

8. Jean Coope and Deborah Roberts, "A Clinic for the Prevention of Osteoporosis in General Practice," *British Journal of General Practice* (July 1990): 295–298.

9. "Osteoporosis: A Woman's Guide," National Osteoporosis Foundation, 1988.

10. Gail A. Greendale, M.D., et al., "Estrogen and Progestin Therapy to Prevent Osteoporosis: Attitudes and Practices of General Internists and Gynecologists," *Journal of General Internal Medicine* 5 (November/December 1990): 464–469.

11. Claus Christiansen, "Hormonal Prevention and Treatment of Osteoporosis—State of the Art 1990," *Journal of Steroid Biochemistry and Molecular Biology* 37, No. 3 (1990): 447–449.

12. Brian E. Henderson, M.D., Annlia Paganini-Hill, Ph.D., and Ronald K. Ross, M.D., "Decreased Mortality in Users of Estrogen Replacement Therapy," *Archives of Internal Medicine* 151 (January 1991): 75–78.

13. Elizabeth Barrett-Connor, M.D., and Trudy L. Bush, Ph.D., M.H.S., "Estrogen and Coronary Heart Disease in Women," *Journal of the American Medical Association* 265, No. 14 (April 10, 1991): 1861–1866.

14. Virginia L. Ernster, Ph.D., et al., "Benefits and Risks of Menopausal Estrogen and/or Progestin Hormone Use," *Preventive Medicine* 17 (1988): 201–223.

15. Ronald K. Ross et al., "Cardiovascular Benefits of Estrogen Replacement Therapy," *American Journal of Obstetrics and Gynecology* (May 1989): 1301–1305.

16. Jane A. Cauley et al., "The Relation of Endogenous Sex Steroid Hormone Concentrations to Serum Lipid and Lipoprotein Levels in Postmenopausal Women," *American Journal of Epidemiology* 132, No. 5 (June 1990): 884–893.

17. ——— et al., "Prevalence and Determinants of Estrogen Replacement Therapy in Elderly Women," *American Journal of Obstetrics and Gynecology* 163, No. 5 (November 1990): 1438–1444.

18. Robin B. Harris, Ph.D., et al., "Are Women Using Postmenopausal Estrogens? A Community Survey," *American Journal of Public Health* 80, No. 10 (October 1990): 1266–1268.

19. Meir J. Stampfer, M.D., et al., "A Prospective Study of Postmenopausal Estrogen Therapy and Coronary Heart Dis-

ease," *New England Journal of Medicine* 313, No. 17 (October 24, 1985): 1044–1049.

CHAPTER FOUR

1. "The Estrogen Question," *Consumer Reports,* September 1991: 587–591.

2. Leif Bergkvist, M.D., et al., "The Risk of Breast Cancer After Estrogen and Estrogen-Progestin Replacement," *The New England Journal of Medicine* 321, No. 5 (August 3, 1989): 293–297.

3. William D. Dupont, Ph.D., and David L. Page, M.D., "Menopausal Estrogen Replacement Therapy and Breast Cancer," *Archives of Internal Medicine* 151 (January 1991): 67–72.

4. Maria Sillero-Arenas, M.D., et al., "Menopausal Hormone Replacement Therapy and Breast Cancer: A Meta-Analysis," *Obstetrics and Gynecology* 79, No. 2 (February 1992): 286–294.

5. Karen K. Steinberg, Ph.D., et al., "A Meta-Analysis of the Effect of Estrogen Replacement Therapy on the Risk of Breast Cancer," *Journal of the American Medical Association* 265, No. 15 (April 17, 1991): 1985–1990.

6. Jennifer L. Kelsey, Ph.D., and Marilie D. Gammon, Ph.D., "The Epidemiology of Breast Cancer," *CA - A Cancer Journal for Clinicians* 41, No. 3 (May/June 1991): 146–165.

7. "Cancer Facts and Figures—1992," American Cancer Society, based on rates from NCI SEER program, 1986–1988.

8. Hans-Olov Adami, M.D., et al., "The Effect of Female Sex Hormones on Cancer Survival," *Journal of the American Medical Association* 263, No. 16 (April 25, 1990): 2189–2193.

9. Brian E. Henderson et al., "Toward the Primary Prevention of Cancer," *Science* 254 (November 22, 1991): 1131–1138.

10. "How to Evaluate Medical News," *UCLA Health Insights* 2, No. 8 (August 1984): 5–6.

11. "Taking Hormones and Women's Health: Choices, Risks and Benefits," a position paper by the National Women's Health Network, Washington, D.C., 8–9.

12. *Dorland's Illustrated Medical Dictionary,* 1596.

CHAPTER FIVE

1. "Estrogen Replacement Therapy," American College of Obstetrics and Gynecology Technical Bulletin 93, June 1986.

2. James W. Long, M.D., *Essential Guide to Prescription Drugs,* 491–494, 655–657.

3. Virginia Burke Karb et al., *Handbook of Drugs for Nursing Practice,* 626–627, 634.

4. *Physicians' Desk Reference,* 1387, 1388, 2510, 2356.

5. R. Don Gambrell, Jr., M.D., "Estrogen Replacement Therapy User Guide" (Dallas: Essential Medical Information Systems, Inc., 1989): 32–56.

CHAPTER SIX

1. Speroff, op. cit., 131.

2. Sadja Greenwood, M.D., "Hormones and Psychology: Is Menopause a Time of Emotional Imbalance?" in *Menopause, Naturally* (Volcano, CA: Volcano Press, 1984).

3. Rosetta Reitz, *Menopause: A Positive Approach* (New York: Penguin Books, 1977): 11–14.

4. Deborah Lott, Gretchen Henkel, and Marvin Karno, M.D., "How to Choose a Psychotherapist," *UCLA Health Insights* (December 1985): 3–4.

5. Winnie Holzman, "Life Class," from MGM Worldwide Television Group's *thirtysomething*, 43–44.

6. Susanne Morgan, *Coping with a Hysterectomy: Your Own Choice, Your Own Solutions* (New York: The Dial Press, 1982): 174.

7. Women's Health Network, 1325 G Street, N.W., Washington, D.C. 20005.

8. Sonia Hamburger, "The Value of the Menopause Clinic: A Personal Opinion," *Maturitas* 12 (1990): 315–317.

9. Myra S. Hunter, "Emotional Well-Being, Sexual Behaviour and Hormone Replacement Therapy," *Maturitas* 12 (1990): 299–314.

10. Barbara B. Sherwin and Barbara E. Suranyi-Cadotte, "Up-Regulatory Effect of Estrogen on Platelet H–Imipramine Binding Sites in Surgically Menopausal Women," *Biology and Psychiatry* 28 (1990): 339–348.

CHAPTER SEVEN

1. Zand, op. cit.

2. Flavia Potenza et al., "Menopause," originally aired on *Feminist Magazine* radio talk show, station KPFK, Los Angeles, California, July 11, 1990.

3. Morgan, op. cit., 169–193.

4. Cathryn Bauer, *Acupressure for Women* (Freedom, California: The Crossing Press, 1988): 110–136.

5. Sachs, op. cit., 113–124.

6. Patricia A. Ladewig, R.N., "Protocol for Estrogen Replacement Therapy in Menopausal Women," *Nurse Practitioner* 10, No. 10 (October 1985): 47.

7. Carlo Gennari and Donato Agnusdei, "Calcitonin, Estrogens and the Bone," *Journal of Steroid Biochemistry and Molecular Biology* 37, No. 3 (1990): 451–455.

8. Marlene Cimons, "U.S. to Test Drug's Ability to Prevent Breast Cancer," *Los Angeles Times,* April 30, 1992: 1, 12.

CHAPTER EIGHT

1. "Are You At Risk? Osteoporosis," National Osteoporosis Foundation, 1991.

2. "Silent Epidemic: The Truth About Women and Heart Disease," American Heart Association, 1989.

3. Stampfer et al., op cit.

4. Bergkvist et al., op cit.

5. Louise A. Brinton, Ph.D., "The Relationship of Exogenous Estrogens to Cancer Risk," *Cancer Detection and Prevention* 7 (1984): 159–171.

6. Henderson et al., op cit.

7. Pamela P. Murray et al., "Oral Contraceptive Use in Women with a Family History of Breast Cancer," *Obstetrics and Gynecology* 73 (1989): 977.

8. Elizabeth Barrett-Connor, M.D., "Postmenopausal Estrogen and Prevention Bias," *Annals of Internal Medicine* 115, No. 6 (September 15, 1991): 455–456.

CHAPTER NINE

1. Gambrell, op. cit., 64–76.

2. Ladewig, op. cit., 45–47.

3. Theodore J. Hahn, M.D., "Early Diagnosis of Osteoporosis," *UCLA Health Insights* 7, No. 4 (April 1989): 2, 6.

4. Editorial, "Should Prescription of Postmenopausal Hormone Therapy Be Based on the Results of Bone Densitometry?" *Annals of Internal Medicine* 113, No. 8 (October 15, 1990): 565–567.

5. Anna N. A. Tosteson et al., "Cost Effectiveness of Screening Perimenopausal White Women for Osteoporosis: Bone Densitometry and Hormone Replacement Therapy," *Annals of Internal Medicine* 113, No. 8 (October 15, 1990): 594–603.

6. "The Estrogen Question," *Consumer Reports.*

Bibliography

. . .

Abrams, Jerome, M.D., M.P.H., "Estrogen Replacement for the 1990s," *New Jersey Medicine* 88, No. 3 (March 1991): 177–179.

Adami, Hans-Olov, M.D., et al., "The Effect of Female Sex Hormones on Cancer Survival," *Journal of the American Medical Association* 263, No. 16, April 25, 1990.

Alfin-Slater, Roslyn B., Ph.D., "How Medicines Affect Your Nutrient Reserves," *UCLA Health Insights* 3, No. 2, February 1985.

American Cancer Society, "Cancer Facts and Figures—1992," based on rates from NCI SEER program, 1986–1988.

American Heart Association, "Silent Epidemic: The Truth About Women and Heart Disease," 1989.

Barrett-Connor, Elizabeth, M.D., "Postmenopausal Estrogen and Prevention Bias," *Annals of Internal Medicine* 115, No. 6, September 15, 1991.

———, and Trudy L. Bush, Ph.D., M.H.S., "Estrogen and Coronary Heart Disease in Women," *Journal of the American Medical Association* 265, No. 14, April 10, 1991.

Bauer, Cathryn, *Acupressure for Women*. Freedom, CA: The Crossing Press, 1988.

Bergkvist, Leif, M.D., et al., "The Risk of Breast Cancer After Estrogen and Estrogen-Progestin Replacement," *The New England Journal of Medicine* 321, No. 5, August 3, 1989.

Brinton, Louise A., Ph.D., "The Relationship of Exogenous Estrogens to Cancer Risk," *Cancer Detection and Prevention* 7, 1984.

Cauley, Jane A., Dr.P.H., et al., "Prevalence and Determinants of Estrogen Replacement Therapy in Elderly Women," *American Journal of Obstetrics and Gynecology* 163, No. 5, November 1990.

————, "The Relation of Endogenous Sex Steroid Hormone Concentrations to Serum Lipid and Lipoprotein Levels in Postmenopausal Women," *American Journal of Epidemiology* 132, No. 5, June 1990.

Christiansen, Claus, "Hormonal Prevention and Treatment of Osteoporosis—State of the Art 1990," *Journal of Steroid Biochemistry and Molecular Biology* 37, No. 3, 1990.

Cimons, Marlene, "U.S. to Test Drug's Ability to Prevent Breast Cancer," *Los Angeles Times,* April 30, 1992.

Clisham, P. R., et al., "Long-Term Transdermal Estradiol Therapy: Effects on Endometrial Histology and Bleeding Patterns," *Obstetrics and Gynecology* 79, February 1992.

Coope, Jean, and Deborah Roberts, "A Clinic for the Prevention of Osteoporosis in General Practice," *British Journal of General Practice,* July 1990.

Dalton, Maureen, "The Menopause," *Gynaecological Endocrinology: A Guide to Understanding and Management.* Oradell, New Jersey: Medical Economics Books, 1989.

Dorland's Illustrated Medical Dictionary, 27th Ed. Philadelphia: W. B. Saunders Co., 1988.

Dupont, William D., Ph.D., and David L. Page, M.D., "Menopausal Estrogen Replacement Therapy and Breast Cancer," *Archives of Internal Medicine* 151, January 1991.

Bibliography

Ernster, Virginia L., Ph.D., et al., "Benefits and Risks of Menopausal Estrogen and/or Progestin Hormone Use," *Preventive Medicine* 17, 1988.

"Estrogen Question, The," *Consumer Reports,* September 1991.

"Estrogen Replacement Therapy," American College of Obstetrics and Gynecology Technical Bulletin 93, June 1986.

"Estrogen Replacement Therapy," *Mayo Clinic Letter,* May 1991.

"Estrogen Use," American College of Obstetrics and Gynecology, Patient Education pamphlet #APO66, May 1986.

Gambrell, R. Don Jr., M.D., *Estrogen Replacement Therapy User Guide.* Dallas: Essential Medical Information Systems, Inc., 1989.

————, "The Menopause—State of the Art in Medicine," *Investigative Radiology* 21 (April 1986): 369–377.

Gennari, Carolo and Donato Agnusdei, "Calcitonin, Estrogens and the Bone," *Journal of Steroid Biochemistry and Molecular Biology* 37, No. 3, 1990.

Gillespy, Thurman III, M.D., and Marjorie P. Gillespy, "Osteoporosis—Metabolic Bone Disease," *Radiologic Clinics of North America* 29, No. 1, January 1991.

Greendale, Gail A., M.D., et al., "Estrogen and Progestin Therapy to Prevent Osteoporosis: Attitudes and Practices of General Internists and Gynecologists," *Journal of General Internal Medicine* 5, November/December 1990.

Greenspan, Francis S., M.D., Ed., "Disorders of the Ovary and Female Reproductive Tract," in *Basic and Clinical Endocrinology.* Norwalk, Connecticut: Appleton & Lange, 1985.

Greenwood, Sadja, M.D., *Menopause, Naturally.* Volcano, CA: Volcano Press, 1984.

205

Hahn, Theodore J., M.D., "Early Diagnosis of Osteoporosis," *UCLA Health Insights* 7, No. 4, April 1989.

Hamburger, Sonia, "The Value of the Menopause Clinic, A Personal Opinion," *Maturitas* 12, 1990.

Harris, Robin B., Ph.D., et al., "Are Women Using Postmenopausal Estrogens? A Community Survey," *American Journal of Public Health* 80, No. 10, October 1990.

Henderson, Brian E., M.D., Annlia Paganini-Hill, Ph.D., and Ronald K. Ross, M.D., "Decreased Mortality in Users of Estrogen Replacement Therapy," *Archives of Internal Medicine* 151, January 1991.

Henderson, Brian E., M.D., et al., "Toward the Primary Prevention of Cancer," *Science* 254, November 22, 1991.

Holzman, Winnie, "Life Class," from MGM Worldwide Television Group's (a Division of MGM-Pathé Communications Co.) *thirtysomething*, 43–44.

"How to Evaluate Medical News," *UCLA Health Insights* 2, No. 8, August 1984.

Hunter, Myra S., "Emotional Well-Being, Sexual Behaviour and Hormone Replacement Therapy," *Maturitas* 12, 1990.

Karb, Virginia Burke, R.N., M.S.N., Sherry F. Queener, Ph.D., and Julia B. Freeman, Ph.D., Eds., *Handbook of Drugs for Nursing Practice*. St. Louis: The C. V. Mosby Company, 1989.

Kase, Lori Miller, "The Mythology of Menopause," *Health*, March 1991.

Kelsey, Jennifer L., Ph.D., and Marilie D. Gammon, Ph.D., "The Epidemiology of Breast Cancer," *CA - A Cancer Journal for Clinicians* 41, No. 3, May/June 1991.

Kohler, Peter O., M.D., and Richard M. Jordan, M.D., Eds., *Clinical Endocrinology*. New York: John Wiley & Sons, 1986.

Ladewig, Patricia A., R.N., "Protocol for Estrogen Replacement Therapy in Menopausal Women," *Nurse Practitioner* 10, No. 10, October 1985.

Long, James W., M.D., *The Essential Guide to Prescription Drugs.* New York: HarperCollins, 1992.

Lott, Deborah, Gretchen Henkel, and Marvin Karno, M.D., "How to Choose a Psychotherapist," *UCLA Health Insights,* December 1985.

Lufkin, Edward G., et al., "Estrogen Replacement Therapy: Current Recommendations," *Mayo Clinic Proceedings* 63, 1988.

Martin, Constance R., Ph.D., "The Female Reproductive System," *Endocrine Physiology.* New York: Oxford University Press, 1985.

Metzger, Deborah A., M.D., Ph.D., and Charles B. Hammond, M.D., "Are Estrogens Indicated for the Treatment of Postmenopausal Women?" *Drug Intelligence and Clinical Pharmacy* 22, June 1988.

Morgan, Susanne, *Coping with a Hysterectomy: Your Own Choice, Your Own Solutions,* New York: The Dial Press, 1982.

Murray, Pamela P., et al., "Oral Contraceptive Use in Women with a Family History of Breast Cancer," *Obstetrics and Gynecology* 73, 1989.

McLachlan, John A., Ed., "Estrogens in the Environment." Raleigh, South Carolina: *Proceedings of the Symposium on Estrogens in the Environment,* September 1979.

Nachtigall, Lila E. and Joan Rattner Heilman, *Estrogen: The Facts Can Change Your Life.* New York: HarperCollins, 1991.

National Institute on Aging, "The Menopause Time of Life," NIH Publication No. 86-2461, Rev. July 1986.

————, "Should You Take Estrogen?" NIH fact sheet, 1988.

National Institute of Arthritis and Musculoskeletal and Skin Diseases, "Osteoporosis: Cause, Treatment, Prevention," NIH Publication 86-2226, Rev. May 1986.

———, "Overview: HHS and Private Sector Efforts in Osteoporosis," 1991.

National Osteoporosis Foundation, "Are You at Risk? Osteoporosis," 1991.

———, "Osteoporosis: A Woman's Guide," 1988.

Physicians' Desk Reference 1992, 46th Ed. Montvale, New Jersey: Medical Economics Data, 1992.

"Postmenopausal Estrogen/Progestin Interventions Trial, The," background paper prepared by Department of Health and Human Services, October 1991.

Potenza, Flavia, et al., "Menopause," originally aired on "Feminist Magazine" radio show, station KPFK, Los Angeles, California, July 11, 1990.

Reitz, Rosetta, *Menopause: A Positive Approach.* New York: Penguin Books, 1977.

Ross, Ronald K., et al., "Cardiovascular Benefits of Estrogen Replacement Therapy," *American Journal of Obstetrics and Gynecology,* May 1989.

Sachs, Judith, *What Women Should Know About Menopause,* New York: Dell Publishing, 1991.

Sherwin, Barbara B. and Barbara E. Suranyi-Cadotte, "Up-Regulatory Effect of Estrogen on Platelet H–Imipramine Binding Sites in Surgically Menopausal Women," *Biology and Psychiatry* 28, 1990.

"Should Prescription of Postmenopausal Hormone Therapy Be Based on the Results of Bone Densitometry?" Editorial, *Annals of Internal Medicine* 113, No. 8, October 15, 1990.

Sillero-Arenas, Maria, M.D., et al., "Menopausal Hormone Replacement Therapy and Breast Cancer: A Meta-Analysis," *Obstetrics and Gynecology* 79, No. 2, February 1992.

Spencer, Greg, Department of Projections, U.S. Census Bureau, April, 1992 interview.

Speroff, Leon, M.D., Robert H. Glass, M.D., and Nathan Kase, M.D., *Clinical Gynecologic Endocrinology and Infertility*, Fourth Ed. Baltimore: Williams & Wilkins, 1989.

Stampfer, Meir J., M.D., et al., "A Prospective Study of Postmenopausal Estrogen Therapy and Coronary Heart Disease," *New England Journal of Medicine* 313, No. 17, October 24, 1985.

Steinberg, Karen K., Ph.D., et al., "A Meta-Analysis of the Effect of Estrogen Replacement Therapy on the Risk of Breast Cancer," *Journal of the American Medical Association* 265, No. 15, April 17, 1991.

"Taking Hormones and Women's Health: Choices, Risks and Benefits," a position paper by the National Women's Health Network, Washington, D.C.

Tosteson, Anna N. A., et al., "Cost Effectiveness of Screening Perimenopausal White Women for Osteoporosis: Bone Densitometry and Hormone Replacement Therapy," *Annals of Internal Medicine* 113, No. 8, October 15, 1990.

"Transdermal Estradiol: A Review," *Drugs* 40, No. 4, 1990.

Turner, C. Donnell, Ph.D., and Joseph T. Bagnara, Ph.D., "Endocrinology of the Ovary," in *General Endocrinology*, Sixth Ed. Philadelphia: W. B. Saunders Co., 1981.

Wolfe, Sidney M., M.D., and Rhoda Donkin Jones, *Women's Health Alert*. Reading, MA: Addison-Wesley Publishing Co., 1991.

Zand, Janet, N.D., O.M.D., "Menopause, A Comfortable Transition," *Delicious!,* November/December 1991.

Index

. . .

217